ABOUT THE AUTHOR

Madeleine Kelly has suffered severe mood disturbance since the age of 16 and was diagnosed ten years later as having a form of manic depression. In the interim she studied medicine at the University of Melbourne but illness forced her withdrawal after five years' effort. She has worked as a casual cleaner, medical secretary, insurance clerk, marketing officer, human resources manager, publicity officer, activist, educator and as a consumer consultant for quality improvement in Victorian public mental health services.

In 1992 Madeleine founded MoodWorks, an education group run by, and for, people with manic depression. She has served as Secretary and President of the Victorian Mental Illness Awareness Council and is a member of the Australian Mental Health Consumers Network, the Disability Employment Action Centre and the Mental Health Legal Centre of Victoria.

Madeleine lives with her husband and children in north-eastern Victoria, where she is pursuing a life in the mainstream while commentating on mental health policy and practice.

LIFE ON A ROLLER-COASTER

LIVING WELL WITH DEPRESSION AND MANIC DEPRESSION

MADELEINE KELLY

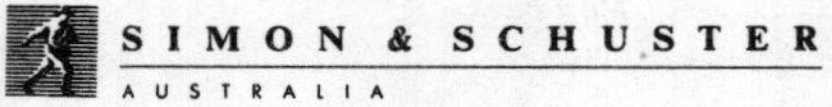
SIMON & SCHUSTER
AUSTRALIA

This book contains the opinions and ideas of its author. It is intended to provide helpful and informative material on the subjects addressed in the book. It is sold with the understanding that the author and publisher are not engaged in rendering medical, health, or any other kind of professional services in the book. The reader should consult his or her medical, health, or other competent professional before adopting any of the suggestions in the book or drawing inferences from it.

The author and publisher disclaim all responsibility for any liability, loss, or risk, personal or otherwise, which is incurred as a consequence, directly or indirectly, of the use and application of any of the contents of this book.

DEDICATION

In memory of Tom Finnigan, 1964 – 1999.
For manic-depressives everywhere and ecclesia dei.

LIFE ON A ROLLER-COASTER
First published in Australia in 2000 by
Simon & Schuster (Australia) Pty Limited
20 Barcoo Street, East Roseville NSW 2069

A Viacom Company
Sydney New York London Toronto Tokyo Singapore

National Library of Australia
Cataloguing-in-Publication data

Kelly, Madeleine, 1959– .
Life on a roller-coaster.

Bibliography.
Includes index.
ISBN 0 7318 0948 3.

1. Manic-depressive illness – Popular works. 2. Depression, Mental – Popular works. I. Title.

616.85/27

Design by Gayna Murphy, Greendot Design
Typesetting by Asset Typesetting Pty Ltd
Set in 11/14 Sabon
Printed in Australia by Griffin Press

10 9 8 7 6 5 4 3 2 1

CONTENTS

ACKNOWLEDGEMENTS

Margaret and Rick Kelly, for teaching me to value making the most of life. Graeme Winterton, Brendan Holwill, Stephen James, for offering me the tools to get out of the mess. David Grounds, for getting behind MoodWorks and everyone at MoodWorks for teaching me how to ride the roller-coaster. Meredith Fuller, Judy Womersley, Jackie Yowell, for giving me the confidence to write. Moira Rayner, for lighting the fire in my belly and public mental health services for providing much of the fuel. All the individuals who allowed me to tell their story, for your generosity to those who read this book. Phil Graley, for travelling with me and challenging how I see the world.

PREFACE

In the early 1990s, I was in hospital because a series of prescription cocktails hadn't lifted my depression. On top of that, I was feeling dreadfully alone, having just been diagnosed as 'manic-depressive'. I thought I was an oddity.

Two weeks earlier, I'd borrowed a book from a classmate from university. When I caught sight of Kate on the ward, I thought she wanted her book back. How had she found out that I was in the loony bin?

She hadn't. She was as embarrassed as I was when we realised we were both patients. 'What are you doing here?' we asked each other in unison.

'Bipolar.' 'Manic depression,' came our respective answers.

I had never met anyone with the same disorder as me. Let alone anyone whom I knew to be totally normal! Embarrassment gave way to relief.

'So you're manic-depressive too?'

'Cool!'

Kate and I made friends with Don, who also has manic depression. Our conversations naturally turned again and again to our common experiences. Kate told us how she sometimes suffered from paranoid ideas when she was severely depressed. Don's eyes lit up—he, too, had had similar experiences, but had never met anyone else who had. In the process of swapping yarns, I noticed that we were giving each other fragments of information about how we managed our lives around our illnesses, and learning more from each other than psychiatry could ever teach.

Not only did we teach each other, we started laughing. At first we laughed at the absurdities of the condition, trading stories of outrageous behaviour. Soon, though, the laughter took on a deeper, healing quality—we laughed at the joy of being fully, comprehensively understood by each other. We laughed together for the joy of discovering from each other how to get the most out of our lives.

Nothing can beat the transforming power of knowledge shared between fellow 'sufferers'. (There are a lot of us around. About three per cent of Australians have recurring mood problems and another two per cent have a single episode of severe depression in their lifetime.) I wanted to share that power to reach ordinary Australians with manic depression and spread the word of our experience and healing laughter.

I want to give readers information and ideas they can use as a starting point in recovering the losses of relationships, jobs, homes, money, credibility, and self-determination that are often sustained through manic depression. Some losses stem from the experience of manic depression in itself. But the more devastating losses occur during treatment and because of the prevailing discriminatory attitudes of society.

This isn't a recipe book—think of it more like the spread of ingredients in front of a television chef. You can select your ingredients to suit yourself and cook a meal to satisfy your own needs and tastes. You won't find absolute prescriptions such as those you've probably already heard: 'Pull your socks up!' 'Take this lithium and you'll feel better.' 'Ask God for forgiveness.' 'Don't stress!' 'Look at all the good things in your life—you've got nothing to be depressed about!'

You won't find many spectacular, embarrassing, bizarre stories in this book because I want to keep the focus on *what we can do to make the most of our lives*. There are many well-written books and articles (though some are simply parasitic voyeurism) on the weird stuff. A number of the more responsible publications are listed at the end of Chapter 1.

When I started out, my main frame of reference was the 'medical model', having experienced and been taught the best of psychiatry's offerings. However, as I interviewed and worked with people who have been treated under psychiatry, I became aware of the dangers posed to human rights when a single paradigm assumes a monopoly on thought, practice, funding and law-making. Nevertheless, I did decide to keep the 'medical model' as the main frame of reference for two reasons. Firstly, I, and many others with manic depression, recognise the benefits that can be derived from medicine. Secondly, it is important to know what psychiatry believes if we are to effectively tackle its worst abuses.

This isn't to say I'm discounting other ways of conceptualising our experience—on the contrary. We can't rebuild whole lives without entertaining ideas from other schools of thought. By considering discrimination, we can deal with stigmatising attitudes. By knowing relevant parts of the law, we can seek justice and minimise the risk of getting into trouble. By using simple psychological tools, we can understand how relationships founder. By looking at our experiences from a spiritual angle, we can see a more complete picture of ourselves and our world.

Whether you adopt a medical approach to your experience or not, there is still the matter of acceptance. Accept, if you like, that you have a medical condition. Better still, accept that you have had problems as a consequence of certain painful experiences that may recur (you don't have to frame it as a life sentence called 'mental illness' or 'manic depression'), and therefore you had better do something about them. But never accept that these experiences must therefore mean a lifetime of submissiveness and loss. If you do that, you're giving up on yourself. There *are* things you can do to have a fulfilled life. You're not responsible for giving yourself this condition, but you, and only you, can take responsible action to make the most of your life as you find it.

I leave it to you to inform yourself and make your own decision about the costs and benefits of treatment, except to say that if you can stay alive long enough, there *will* be a time when you can rebuild *and it will be worth it.* If this means taking medicine or going to hospital, even if you don't want to, do it.

I have written, as much as I have been able, from a 'consumer's perspective'. I have tried to relate people's experiences as if they are speaking directly to the reader. In doing so, one of the challenges has been to identify my own biases and blinkers, my own lack of insight-born-of-experience and to try not to put a third-person spin on any of the experiences I've conveyed. I wasn't confident of being able to tell some stories without bias, in particular the experiences of gays, lesbians, indigenous people, people in the forensic system, people whose experience with drugs or alcohol is clearer to them than mine is to me and people from other religious backgrounds from mine. May the healing power and wisdom of your stories emerge in your way, in your time.

On the subject of story telling, let me make a few comments about language. The language we use can have subtle but damaging effects. I have a strong preference for the term 'medicine' over 'medication'. 'Medicine' means 'the science or practice of the diagnosis and treatment of illness and injury and the preservation of health' and *'a substance or preparation used in the treatment of illness.'*[1] (My italics.) 'Medication', however, means 'the action of treating medically; treatment with a medicinal substance.'[2] But in the middle of the twentieth century a new meaning crept in: 'a drug or drugs prescribed or given as medical treatment.'[3] The effect of this new meaning for 'medication' is subtle but potent: the terms 'medicine' and 'medication' are now used interchangeably as if there is no distinction between the terms. But there is an enormous distinction. If I 'take my medicine' I am taking action myself. If I 'take my medication', I am submitting to the action of the doctor or nurse who is medicating me. The term 'medication' carries the expectation of passiveness on my part.

Another disconcerting effect of language is the change in the name of manic depression. Psychiatry has tried to persuade us that the 'correct' term for our condition is 'bipolar affective disorder'. I reject 'bipolar' as a term, not only because it is someone else's term for our experience, and not only because most members of the public haven't a clue what it means (which sets back community education immensely), but also because it is insufficiently descriptive of the experience of the condition. 'Bipolar' refers to two poles of mood, yet the condition is about variations in three elements: mood, activity and thinking.

The older terms of melancholia and mania are much more poignant and meaningful, and they carry some history, some reference point, in the minds of the public. A cold is still 'a cold', epilepsy is still 'epilepsy'; schizophrenia has been 'schizophrenia' since 1911,[4] but manic depression has only been 'bipolar' for twenty years or so.[5] Why should we have to cower behind a term, defined by others, that applies only to some of us, denies the public knowledge that our experience is common, and disconnects us from the history of those who have had similar experiences?

I cringe when I hear someone say (unless with humour or pride) 'I'm a manic-depressive'. The same goes for 'I'm a diabetic', 'I'm a schizophrenic', 'I'm an asthmatic' and 'I'm an epileptic'. Apart from the fact that it's poor grammar to use an adjective when a noun is called for, it implies that the person is giving me permission to think of him or her as being nothing other than their condition.

The first seven chapters of this book give details of the medical approach to manic depression, the treatment available and the law relating to having treatment of a mental illness.

Chapter 8 deals with the period immediately following a crisis. In Chapter 9 I introduce a step-by-step method of limiting and preventing damage from recurring episodes. You can follow the steps in detail if you like or use them to prompt your own ideas for dealing with your experiences—feel free to adapt the steps. The chapters that follow give information and ideas about education and employment (Chapter 10), money (Chapter 11), adult relationships (Chapter 12), children (Chapter 13) and spirituality (Chapter 14).

Readers who don't have manic depression will learn much by reading between the lines—through a glimpse from our perspective you might revise the role you play as a 'carer', or develop a new angle to psycho-education or research if you're a mental health professional.

I have quoted from many people with manic depression and I am deeply grateful for their generosity in sharing their experiences, observations and wisdom. Most have given me explicit consent to quote them. Otherwise pseudonyms have been used to protect people from discrimination. Where ideas have been expressed by more than one person and where I was unable to contact the person to ask for their consent, I have fictionalised their story or 'quote'.

Everyone who has contributed to this book joins me, I am sure, in wishing readers the roller-coaster ride of a lifetime.

INTRODUCTION

When things start to go haywire, let's face it—it's scary. Questions flood in: What's wrong with me? Why am I so miserable? Why can't I get out of bed? Why can't I concentrate at work? Why am I so grumpy? Why are people telling me to calm down? I drink too much but I can't not drink and I don't know why. Why can't I sleep?

We supply answers: 'It must be me. I'll just have to look on the bright side.' 'I'm not hyped up, I'm just busy—look at how much work I'm doing!' 'This is all so-and-so's fault.'

Things improve and life goes on. Then it happens again, and the questions flood back. Sooner or later the pattern repeats and we begin to wonder if life will ever be smooth again. Nevertheless we battle on.

For some of us the pain eventually escalates. Or we lose something important—a job, a relationship, a good credit rating. We crash into a crisis of confidence. Spurred by panic that we might lose everything, even life itself, we redouble our efforts to keep on an even keel. We might cast around for a better diet, better relationship, better job, better place to live, less stress, natural healing, relief with drugs or alcohol.

The last port of call for many is psychiatry; after all who wants to have to admit they might be crazy? The unlucky ones don't get to choose who helps them when they're carted off to hospital against their wishes.

Whether you've chosen psychiatry, or psychiatry and the

law have chosen you, you'll be asked to view your experiences as a 'sickness'—a mental illness called manic depression. If you were plagued with unanswerable questions before, now utter chaos sets in. 'I can't be crazy!' You'll be offered an explanation for your experiences based on the idea that you are sick, and persuaded to take medicine to 'get well again'.

So you take it. And things improve, life goes on. Phew! Or things don't improve. You might even get worse. Then you despair. You accept the line that you're sick and you try other doctors, other medicines until you either get better or you're sedated off your face. Or you reject the idea of illness and go back to your old ways of coping.

Although manic depression is serious and ongoing, it is intermittent and there are good prospects for medical control of symptoms. But before we bring the illness under control our education may have been disrupted; our marriages stretched; our work and careers interrupted; our law-abiding natures temporarily changed and our financial situation in chaos.

This is the roller-coaster ride. Welcome aboard!

I don't want to try to persuade anyone who's on the roller-coaster that they can turn the clock back to when things were 'normal' (if they ever were normal). And I'd be lying outright if I said I could offer you techniques that will ensure you never get depressed or high again. But what I do know is how much better life can be if you never accept that you'll be sick, miserable, out of control, incompetent and dependent forever.

Breaking out from despair is difficult; freeing yourself from messages that encourage you to give up takes superhuman effort. But it's your life, and there are things you can do to make the most of it. If you can't believe I'm serious, that's okay—humour me. You might think my experiences must be less damaging than yours are and therefore my ideas won't be useful to you. I don't pretend to be the person who has suffered the most, or the least, from manic depression but I simply offer my own and other people's experiences. So, if you're game to try a bit of self-help, let me ride with you for a while.

1

WHAT IS 'MANIC DEPRESSION'?

I many times thought peace had come,
When peace was far away…
Emily Dickinson

Manic depression is a painful, recurring pattern of variation of exaggerated mood, activity and thinking that causes damage to one or more important aspects of life. The pain can be relieved or prevented with psychiatric medicines and the potential damage limited by the sufferer. Manic depression is thought to confer on some sufferers the capacity for greatness in the arts, literature and leadership.

The experiences of manic depression can be roughly grouped into three states: mania, depression and wellness.

MANIA AND HYPOMANIA

Also called 'high', mania is a dangerous state of extreme elation along with hyperactivity and fast or otherwise altered thinking. Mania is at the extreme end of the scale while hypomania (literally 'little mania') is milder. Sometimes, but not always, hypomania can escalate into mania.

Carole described a manic episode to me:

I don't remember how long I'd been on this high and I was pretty high, actually. I was in hospital and I remember the night nurse came around in a very colourful dress.

The dress became like it was alive—really glistening and the colours were really exaggerated and beautiful. The next day I started cleaning out the clothes that I'd brought to hospital—and I can't remember why—but I was doing a lot of things, going from one thing to another. I got this idea that I had to purify myself. So I started cleaning everything out. I started throwing out all my makeup. I threw out my hairbrushes—I was going to use my fingers to comb my hair. I threw out the tissues because I wasn't going to cry anymore. Just anything and everything. Then I had a shower. I completely changed my hospital bed.

My parents had come in to visit with flowers and the sheepskin I used for my sore back. I wrapped the flowers in the sheepskin and went and threw them in the rubbish bin —in a symbolic way . That was a very symbolic time—everything I was doing was very symbolic. So I walked down the street and threw 'Mum and Dad' in the rubbish bin.

...And then I went and had a shower and I threw out all my soap and everything. Now I only had Velvet soap which was pure. I had a shower, and washed my hair. I washed myself, scrubbed myself up and then got out of the shower and then I was feeling really thirsty. I couldn't use a glass so I had to use my hand like Jesus so I was drinking with my cupped hand.

Let's tease out the elements that go to make up mania—mood, activity and thinking.

Mood

Hypomania can be bliss. We have a high level of self-confidence, a positive outlook on the world and our own prospects. Anything is possible. We have largesse. Others, swayed by us, feed from our ebullience. Such a good feeling makes us reluctant to notice if we are escalating into mania.

Elation is the key mood of mania although it may not always be present. Along with elation are supreme self-confidence, a sense of purpose, even a calling. Everything is larger than life. We are invincible—utterly. Others call us grandiose. They tell us to slow down; there is fear in their eyes; we get incredibly frustrated with them as they cannot keep up with us. We become spiritual—even non-Christians find themselves in a church during mania, overwhelmed with the mystery and majesty of religious icons and spaces. We have a mission and there is no time to lose. Carole continues her story:

And then I got dressed up in all my clean clothes, signed out for a walk and rolled along to St. Mary's. When I got there all the lights and everything—the statues—everything was really glittering at me, like really strong lighting, jumping at me. What time of day was this? I think it was the late afternoon. I think I was going to go and take communion.

All these lights were really dazzling me and I fainted and the next minute I was out in the vestry with all these people trying to get me to come to.

Many times when I was on a high I did go to St. Mary's. I'm not Catholic but I was sort of brought up as a Catholic. The whole thing was so beautiful—I was sitting there crying and all these nuns were concerned. I wasn't crying because I was sad, I was crying because it was so beautiful. That actually happened in another church too, I went to church at Easter time. I fainted—everything was so beautiful—it overwhelms you, I suppose you'd say.

Activity

In hypomania, we get lots done, whatever our field. Sleep becomes less important. Rachel's painting becomes confident and ambitious when she's a little high:

You get an awful lot achieved. My painting... If you go off on a tangent and you're doing something you particularly want to finish, if you're slightly manic you get it done an awful lot quicker than if you're not...

I started this 6-by-4-foot canvas eighteen months ago—but the hypomania ran out before I finished it.

As hypomania starts to escalate into mania, we talk to our friends on the phone—twenty calls in an evening is not unheard of. We don't sleep, we can't sleep and we don't want to because we have so much to do. We write poetry all through the night. We talk at the rate of a speeded-up film. We paint, draw, sew. We do extraordinary things, outrageous things, unlawful things. We might want to bonk everything in sight—and sometimes do—all to no satisfaction. We drink a lot. A helluva lot. We spend our money. We spend the bank's money. We spend our friends' money. We buy three cars and $5,000 worth of clothing. Or take out a loan for $300,000 to buy shares in a newly listed gold mining venture.

Thinking

We can make people laugh—we're the life of the party. We can't stop 'contributing' to class; jokes and puns keep popping into our brains.

I felt a clearing in my mind
As if my brain had split;
I tried to match it, seam by seam,
But could not make them fit.

The thought behind I strove to join
Unto the thought before,
But sequence ravelled out of reach
Like balls upon a floor.

Emily Dickinson

As mania approaches, we can't stop seeing connections between obscure things. We have brilliant ideas in business, literature, finance, farming, politics, religion, then we link them up in a grand unifying theory which we forget by next week. We are irresistibly persuasive. As mania escalates, we might see things that aren't there and be terrified. We might believe we are the Virgin Mary, Jesus Christ or the Devil. Elation becomes confusion, which gives way to chaos.

Thinking in hypomania is clearer, more incisive, more creative than we were before the hypomania started. We are personable and witty without being indecipherable. Rachel told me:

> You're up there. You can answer every question on 'Sale of the Century'. You're on this little journey on the borderline where nothing can hurt you, nothing can harm you and you have a great old time.

During hypomania, the thought disorder isn't really off the beam and many of us carry out brilliant work, like Jonathan, who published fifteen academic research papers in as many years.

The process of thinking during mania has been compared to the process of creative writing. In one study, it was found that writers and people in a manic phase consider more ideas and concepts, and sort and categorise ideas more, and in more unusual ways, than other people.[1]

DEPRESSION

Mood

Everything is grey; the colour has seeped out of everything around us. Nothing matters much at all. We wake and feel the millstone thudding on our chests. We'd shrug our shoulders if we could be bothered. Depression is 'lessness'—pointlessness, hopelessness, haplessness, helplessness.[2] Even angerlessness unless we are irritable, in which case we have tolerancelessness. In deep depression we have emotionlessness.

Carole describes the 'lessness':

For about twelve months I used to say I had lost my feelings. I couldn't feel anything. If somebody that I love or one of my family members had've got run over in front of me, I wouldn't have reacted. I used to describe it as being a shell of a person—everything inside of me died and I had just my physical body that I was walking around in. It's total emotional shutdown. My face was like a mask. It had no expression.

Activity

We prefer to, and sometimes do, spend days on end in bed. We don't go out. We let the answering machine take all the calls, and then we don't ring people back. We don't eat, we lose weight. We don't shower and we wear yesterday's clothes for a week. We don't read to the children, or take them to the park or help with homework. Writer Jan Stumbles put it this way:

The skills, ease of movement, expressions on the face...all become locked.

Locked up, away, out of reach of their owner, much less anybody else, so that finally, even walking is awkward...If you can no longer move, speak, think, but can only grit your teeth and wait, ride the waiting, then possibility is fully exorcised, perhaps banished.[3]

Thinking

Mild depression can leave us unable to concentrate or have difficulty making otherwise-easy decisions.

In severe depression, it's as if your brain has seized up. If you can think at all, you might think: 'I can't do anything.' Which is probably true at this point! You might go on: 'Therefore I'm not pulling my weight in this family/organisation. I won't ever feel any better because I've felt this way for so long. So I'm a burden on everyone. Not only can I not do anything, I'm bad, irretrievably bad. So I should kill myself.'

There might be paranoia as well. Stephen told me, 'I can tell I'm getting depressed when I start suspecting that people at work are trying to sabotage my projects.'

MIXED STATES

Mixed states occur where some symptoms of depression are mixed with symptoms of mania. Between 40 per cent and 48 per cent of people with Bipolar Disorder have 'mixed' symptoms.[4] Given this, it is no wonder that many of us feel we don't really fit the descriptions in the books, or that none of it applies to us and they must have the diagnosis wrong.

WELLNESS

After gradually recovering from months or years of illness, it's sometimes difficult for us and those around us to identify when we are well. As Mary observed:

> Once people become aware that you are 'a manic-depressive', they simply will not allow you to have a bad day. Only 'normal' people are allowed to have 'bad days'. If a 'manic-depressive' has a day that is worse than average, we're not allowed to write it off as a 'bad day'. Carers latch onto the tiniest thing and before you know it they're ringing the psychiatrist.

When we're well, most days are easy to cope with. We can plan, we can socialise and do everything that others take for granted but it is important to recognise that wellness includes having an 'ordinary' bad day and an 'ordinary' good day from time to time.

Once a lengthy period of wellness has been established, we can enjoy a sunrise with neither dread of the day nor terrifying elation. And we might say 'Thank you' to whomever: Lithium, or God, or Dr X, or Fate. And pat ourselves on the back every time we experience something for what it is.

Mood

When we are well, we don't really notice our moods. Neither suicidal nor supremely self-confident, we are able to just get on with the business of living. We may have ups and downs that are a little larger than everyone else's but are manageable nonetheless.

Activity

We sleep regularly. We participate in family life and we can put in a good day's work. We don't get as much done as we did if we were hypomanic and this is often a source of frustration. Our ups and downs might bother us if we notice that our output at work or at home goes in fits and starts—but it's nothing like the lurching ship of a major episode.

Thinking

We notice that others are neither afraid of us nor trying to cheer us up. If we've been hypomanic before, we grieve for the loss of intellectual or creative power. We can tell we're well because our thoughts are neither running away into chaos nor bogged in mallee dust.

STAGES OF THE ROLLER-COASTER JOURNEY

Crisis and diagnosis

The period between the starting of symptoms, which can be as early as childhood or teenage years, and being accurately diagnosed with manic depression can be ten or more years. During this time we may be misdiagnosed as having schizophrenia, sentenced by the courts as delinquents or simply left to battle on alone. If we know a bit about manic depression, we just might be able to be appropriately diagnosed and treated earlier. The diagnosis, when it comes, can create a variety of reactions.

Jonathan felt he was 'in business' when he received his diagnosis.

I felt good, because I felt that I was in safe hands and that Dr Z would know what to do.

By the time she was diagnosed, Mary had been so messed around that she didn't care.

He kept telling me that he thought it was bipolar. It didn't really mean anything because I'd been told 'You're a paranoid schizophrenic and anorexic and depressive'—yeah, yeah.

Carole felt that the diagnosis offered some hope for treatment.

I didn't know what was wrong with me for that eighteen months. I'd been on lots of different tablets and I felt I was never getting better so when I was actually given the label I felt that there was now some hope of treatment for my illness.

In my own case, my scientific mind had been researching at every opportunity. I had learned about manic depression in medical school. I also learned that lithium, a naturally occurring rock salt, is used for treatment. Wondering if it occurred in natural mineral waters, I scoured the shelves of the supermarket one day for mineral water that listed lithium as an ingredient. There are some, but in such minute concentrations I would have had to drink gallons of water a day. When I was finally diagnosed, I was horrified at having a 'mental illness' label but I was quite chuffed at having got the diagnosis right!

Emerging from crisis

You could be forgiven for thinking that once you've been diagnosed, life should return to normal fairly promptly—you get sick, you go to the doctor and get a cure. However, finding effective medicine can take even the most astute treatment team some time to work out. More damaging, for many of us, is the blame and shame that are the social consequences of this and other mental illnesses.

Damage prevention

In the meantime, we realise that the combination of the condition, the treatment and the social consequences present us with a long-term challenge.

Carole describes how she rose to the challenge.

This is my fifteenth year with manic depression.
Sometimes with depression I can go to bed feeling all right and can wake up in the morning feeling rock bottom. Other times I tend to recognise the signs of depression—not sleeping, waking up early in the morning, not wanting to eat, being irritable. Over the past years I think I recognise depression more than the highs, and act on it more quickly. I make a plan that if I don't feel better in four days I'll contact my psychiatrist. It's the same with highs. If I start getting overactive, especially talkative, I really try to quieten myself.

Now that I have acceptance I'm much more in tune with what I want to do. I like to be free...and I like to continually learn about my illness. I'm more in control now than I've ever been in the past.

If things go wrong mood-wise—if I'm depressed—I just try to stay with it and not get too bogged down by the fact that I'm feeling down. Sometimes I get very excitable and I don't know whether it's going to grow into a high and I've got to try and slow down and calm down. I'll go up and get a video and make myself sit and watch it.

Notice how effortlessly Carole seems to monitor her mood state and her dispassionate way of dealing with it. Plans like

Carole's and the ability to judge when we need help from another person are the keys to improving our quality of life.

Recovering quality of life

At some stage, we reach a point where we can start to actively plan to improve the quality of our lives. We are making headway again in some areas, yet we are prepared for setbacks. We are confident that disaster is a thing of the past because we are now prepared. We maintain control over symptoms—in short, we're living with it. As Jonathan says, 'Jonathan includes his manic depression.' While manic depression is still a significant part of your life, it no longer dominates.

We can see the horizon again. Day-to-day mood variations or exaggerated premenstrual symptoms might persist. We might be coping also with the consequences of previous disasters—money, people or jobs. We might be tolerating unwanted effects of medicine. But over time we become productive again, we can see our purpose once more and we no longer live in terror of the swinging monster.

Time, information and experience will tell us how to minimise the impact of manic depression. A bit of plain gutsiness will allow us to accept that manic depression is part of our life. An adventurous spirit will allow us to recover the many losses we sustained and to 'get a life'. This book aims to pass on information and experience. It's up to you to supply the guts and the adventure.

2

SAY THAT LAST BIT AGAIN? MEDICAL INFORMATION

It can be difficult to grasp what medical professionals are talking about at the best of times, especially if your memory and concentration are limited by symptoms, medicine or life trauma. This chapter gives you a rundown of medical information, so you can consider it when your head space clears.

I've included a 'Jargon Decoder' (Appendix I), which is a glossary of terms you'll come across in this book and in talking with mental health professionals.

One word of warning: sometimes when reading about a medical condition, we can persuade ourselves that we have its symptoms. This is a common phenomenon amongst medical students who develop 'symptoms' of the very disease they are currently studying! Use this chapter for information about your own experience rather than to diagnose yourself.

TYPES OF MANIC DEPRESSION

Manic depression has been defined and redefined by the psychiatric profession over the years. The definitions currently in use in Australia are taken from 'DSM-IV', the *Diagnostic and Statistical Manual of Mental Disorders*[1] Fourth Edition, published by the American Psychiatric Association. This manual lists various criteria that a person's illness must meet in order to be diagnosed. The criteria include:

- whether an episode of mood disturbance has occurred in the past;
- whether that episode was depressive, manic, hypomanic or mixed; and
- making sure the condition *is* a mood disorder and not something else.

The criteria have been developed for the use of researchers (so they can 'compare apples with apples'), and mental health workers (so they know what each other is talking about).

There are five major categories of mood disorder that together make up the 'manic-depressive spectrum':

- Bipolar Affective Disorder Type I;
- Major Depressive Disorder;
- Bipolar Affective Disorder Type II;
- Cyclothymia; and
- Dysthymic Disorder.

Technically, the term 'bipolar' only covers Bipolar I and Bipolar II Disorders. These five categories, while being different from each other in many ways, can all be self-managed by sufferers, using techniques discussed in this book. For ease of reference, I'll use the term 'manic depression' unless I'm specifically referring to one or more of the categories.

Bipolar Affective Disorder Type I

This is what most people think of as manic depression. To get diagnosed you need to have had at least one manic episode or one mixed episode. Over the course of the illness, it's likely you'll also have depressive episodes.

Bipolar I affects about equal numbers of men and women. Women with Bipolar I have an increased risk of having a mood episode around childbirth, and the premenstrual part of the cycle can certainly worsen a current episode of mania, hypomania, mixed state or depression.

Major Depressive Disorder

Major Depressive Disorder involves episodic severe depression but you don't get hypomania or mania. If you have one episode of Major Depression, you have a 50 per cent chance of having another. If you have a second episode, your chances of having another increase to around 70 per cent. If you are unlucky enough to have a third episode, you have a 90 per cent chance of yet another.[2] In between episodes people recovery fully or partially.

Sometimes people go on to experience hypomanic or manic episodes—if that happens, you are awarded a new diagnosis of Bipolar Disorder.

Bipolar Affective Disorder Type II

Bipolar II involves Major Depressive episodes on a recurring basis, with recurring hypomanic episodes, but no full-blown mania.

To get diagnosed you need to have had at least one Major Depressive episode and at least one hypomanic episode. Once you have a manic or a mixed episode, the diagnosis changes to Bipolar I.

Up to 70 per cent of hypomanic episodes happen just before or just after a depressive episode. Rapid cycling (four or more episodes in a year) occurs in about 10–15 per cent of people with Bipolar II. Ultra-rapid cycling can also occur, with more frequent fluctuations.

Women with Bipolar II have an increased risk of having an episode related to reproductive events.

Cyclothymia

Cyclothymia gives you hypomania and mild depression. You may develop Bipolar I as well as Cyclothymia. The likelihood of this is around 15–50 per cent.[3]

While not as spectacularly devastating as Bipolar I, II or Major Depressive Disorders, Cyclothymia can still cause significant damage to work, education, employment and relationships.

Dysthymic Disorder

Dysthymic Disorder is a seemingly never-ending, grumbling, pain-in-the-neck sense of being mildly depressed but not so depressed as to be in desperate or suicidal pain. The main criterion for diagnosis is that we are chronically[4] depressed—most of the day, every day, for at least two years, with no more than two months free of the depression.

Other terms for mood disorders

To add confusion, there are a number of other terms still in use that you'll hear to describe mood disorders. Here are some of them.

Unipolar depression This is roughly equivalent to Major Depressive Disorder. So called from *uni*, one and *polar*, pole—that is, the mood shifts towards only the depressive 'pole'.

Seasonal affective disorder An older term for a variant of manic depression that tends to recur in winter.

Post-natal depression Another older term that describes the major depressive episode experienced by some women after giving birth. Post-natal depression has been swallowed up by the DSM-IV definition of the other mood disorders with the addition of 'With Postpartum Onset'.[5] In other words, you can have 'Major Depressive Disorder with Postpartum Onset' or 'Bipolar I Disorder with Postpartum Onset' and so on.

I'd be sad to see the term post-natal depression fall out of use because campaigns to increase public awareness of the relationship of childbirth with mood disorder has increased community acceptance of sufferers of a severe, life-threatening illness who, in the past, have been subject to shame and discrimination.

Reactive depression As far as terminology goes, reactive depression is an oldie but a goodie to hang on to.

Reactive depression is getting depressed *because of* something—compared with depression that has no apparent cause. One of my mentors, Dr David Grounds, calls it 'Collingwood supporters' depression' to describe the poor beggars who followed Collingwood before 1990 in the Australian Football League. (Before they won the premiership in 1990, Collingwood often made it to the finals but always managed to lose. They put it down to the 'colliwobbles' and their supporters were always devastated—'reactive depression'!)

Although DSM-IV doesn't make a distinction between Major Depressive Disorder that is reactive and Major Depressive Disorder that comes out of the blue, it's something to keep in mind when you're considering treatment options. One form of treatment, cognitive behavioural therapy, is especially effective for the reactive aspects of depression. (See Chapter 5.)

OTHER CONDITIONS

Schizophrenia

The most well-known and highly publicised mental illness, schizophrenia is a 'progressive' illness. It's a disorder of thought and perception that gradually, insidiously erodes your ability to do things as well as you used to, despite the effectiveness of antipsychotic medicine that keeps you inside reality.

Schizophrenia is *not* a 'split personality', no matter how often your neighbour might tell you it is.

Schizophrenia is primarily a disorder of thought, in comparison with manic-depressive illness, which is primarily a disorder of mood. However, the two conditions share a propensity for psychotic episodes which may include hallucinations and delusions. Manic-depressive illness tends to give us delusions based on either elated or depressed themes, for example, believing you're the Virgin Mary, or the management guru of the millennium, or that your family has decided you'd be better off dead. On the other hand, delusions in schizophrenia tend to be less well understood by non-sufferers, for example, believing there are messages for you in the number plates of cars.

Thought disorders occur in both conditions but there are a number of key differences. Manic thinking is easily derailed, distracted, tangential and playful, with fast, emphatic speech patterns, while it is thought that 'poverty of speech', 'autistic' thinking and 'absurdity' are features of schizophrenia.[6]

Schizophrenia is readily treated with antipsychotic agents which, unfortunately, do have their downsides.

Schizo-affective disorder

Sometimes mania can be difficult for psychiatrists to distinguish from the psychosis of schizophrenia. Either there are two sorts of psychosis or there is one sort of psychosis with different aspects to it. As long ago as 1933 a 'continuum' was proposed by researchers, which puts schizophrenic-type (thinking) psychosis at one end, affective-type (mood) psychosis at the other, and a hybrid 'schizo-affective' psychosis in the middle.[7]

While debate among scientists continues, the main issue for us is whether we are getting the most appropriate treatment. Generally, schizophrenic symptoms are known to respond best to antipsychotic agents, while manic-depressive symptoms respond best to mood stabilisers (for example, lithium and anticonvulsants). Regardless of the existence or otherwise of a 'schizo-affective disorder', we need to be accurately diagnosed and treated according to our symptoms and signs.

Drug-induced psychosis

This is a psychotic condition caused by the use of illegal drugs such as amphetamines and hallucinogens. It is thought that marijuana can trigger an episode of psychosis in a vulnerable person.[8]

Anxiety conditions

Anxiety conditions comprise a wide variety of disorders: phobias, panic disorders and obsessive-compulsive disorder. Obsessive-Compulsive Disorder (OCD) is a type of anxiety disorder featuring repetitive thoughts (obsessions) and behaviours (compulsions). It can be, but doesn't have to be, associated with manic-depressive illness, with researchers exploring possible similarities in alterations to neurotransmitters in both conditions.[9]

Borderline personality disorder

An antiquated term originally meaning 'bordering on the psychotic', this is a developmental disorder of the 'self', causing individuals to be unsure of their identity, beliefs and values. Along with mood shifts, people with borderline can have unstable relationships and impulsive, self-destructive behaviour, high anger levels and feelings of abandonment and emptiness. Borderline is 'a pervasive pattern of instability of mood, interpersonal relationships, and self-image, beginning by early adulthood'.[10] Some psychiatrists believe it is a mood disorder modified by sexual or other abuse.

Eating disorders

Anorexia nervosa is characterised by 'self-induced weight loss, intense fear of becoming fat and cessation of periods'. In bulimia nervosa, there are 'repeated bouts of uncontrolled overeating, an intense fear of gaining weight and attempts to limit its increase through extreme weight control strategies'.[11]

From a practical point of view, anorexia (which literally means 'no appetite') is a classic symptom of major depression—and one that can lead to misdiagnosis.

Conditions that often occur with manic depression

As if bipolar is not difficult enough, many people suffer also from other conditions. Alcoholism is prevalent among people with manic depression—and mood disorders are prevalent among people who abuse or are dependent on alcohol. Similarly, users of illicit drugs, particularly cocaine, are up to thirty times more likely than the general population to have a mood disorder.[12]

My great-grandfather is said to have been an alcoholic. He is quoted down the family tree as having said 'I drink to still the mind'. I can understand exactly what he meant by that: alcohol does counter the mind's racing restlessness in hypomania and mania, but its consequences can be as bad or worse than the consequences of the mood disorder.

Other people have to contend with conditions such as the aftermath of sexual abuse and/or lack of support or even hostility from family members and difficulties in intimate relationships. These issues can trigger and overlap with both borderline personality disorder and manic depression.

Some people who have acquired brain damage, certain cancers, multiple sclerosis and metabolic conditions also develop mood disorder. Manic and depressive symptoms are common in people with HIV/AIDS where the infection has reached the central nervous system. The symptoms are often, but not always, part of an overall degenerative condition ('AIDS dementia') involving the whole nervous system.

Epilepsy, too, often overlaps with manic depression—whether they are two separate conditions occurring in an individual or whether each is an aspect of a single disease process is still being researched and debated. Similarly, there are more people with both manic depression and borderline personality disorder than would be expected by chance alone.[13]

This is an area of research that is not yet clear. But it is not surprising for an individual to suffer from more than one of the following: manic depression, epilepsy, alcoholism, borderline personality disorder or childhood sexual abuse.

WHO SUFFERS FROM MANIC DEPRESSION?

Of the five types of mood disorder, mean prevalence rates are available for Bipolar I Disorder (1.2 per cent) and Major Depression (4.4 per cent).[14]

This equates with 220,000 individuals in Australia with Bipolar I Disorder and another 807,000 with Major Depression,[15] a total of more than one million people.

Of course, many people are not diagnosed and some will never come to the attention of medical services. Many find that they can live with their periodic difficulties. Others camouflage their mood problems with drug or alcohol abuse and may not recognise themselves to be suffering a mood disorder.

Bipolar Affective Disorder appears to affect men and women roughly equally. Major Depression affects more women than men.

Because of problems with methodology, it is difficult to compare how common manic depression is between single and married people or between cultures, race and social class, although there is some evidence suggesting that the bipolar category of manic depression may be more prevalent in upper socioeconomic classes.[16]

EPISODES AND CYCLES

Jonathan told me:

> I went through university failing every odd year, which was '65, '67 and '69 and yet I even took out the Exhibition, which was first-class Honours, in the even years. So this shows it can be plotted as a results graph versus time that I have had a two-year cycle of mood swings ... Since I've been treated with lithium, this cycle seems to have gone away.

Robert Schumann, the composer, had manic depression. Most of his significant works were written 'on the way up'—in periods of hypomania. Not surprisingly, there were long periods in which he wrote little, and these are said to have equated with periods of depression.[17] Of course, Schumann didn't have access to treatment, and Jonathan wasn't diagnosed or treated until after his university years. Cycles are much easier to identify if the illness is untreated.

Manic depression doesn't always stick to the calendar in the early years, but over a longer period of time the rhythm and beat of the condition can become clearer.

Episodes usually last the same length of time in each individual. Over the first three to five episodes, the period between episodes becomes shorter. After this, the symptom-free period settles down and becomes more predictable.[18] Manic episodes tend to be shorter and start more suddenly than episodes of depression.[19]

Cycle patterns

Do you go high and then crash, or the other way around? There are some gender differences in cycle patterns. For example, women are more likely to cycle from mania to depression—men are just as likely to move from mania to depression as from depression to mania.[20]

There hasn't been an enormous amount of scientific work on the issue of patterns. One question that has been researched is the extent to which episodes consist of a single mood shift, or two or more mood shifts in opposite directions. It appears from three studies that 50–70 per cent of episodes of mania or depression are single-direction episodes, that is only mania or depression. Dual-direction episodes make up most of the remainder.

If we had a room full of people with Bipolar Disorder, what would we expect to find as their experience of mania and/or depression? A study conducted in 1987[21] looked at mood cycles. The researchers divided people into three groups according to their psychiatric history:

- severe depression and severe mania 'MD'
- severe mania with mild depression 'Md'
- severe depression with hypomania 'Dm'

The following table reveals their findings:

Pattern of illness	Men (%)	Women (%)
MD—mania and depression	45	35
Md—mania and mild depression	22	10
Dm—depression and hypomania	23	55

Table 2.1 Illness patterns in Bipolar Disorder. Adapted from Angst, 1987[22]

Between episodes

Manic depression is characterised by its ability to resolve completely, only to return after some time. Of course, this is significantly modified by medicine and most people taking medicine don't have major recurrences. For an unlucky few individuals, symptoms may only partially resolve after an episode of major depression.[23] For others, the unwanted effects of medicine can limit how healthy they are in between episodes.

SEVERITY

The severity of each episode can vary between individuals, as well as within one individual over time. Of course, effective treatment can limit and even eliminate symptoms.

TREATABILITY

Manic depression responds to medicine such as mood stabilisers and antidepressants. Sometimes antipsychotic agents or tranquillisers are also used. More details are given in Chapter 4.

MEDICAL THEORIES OF CAUSE

The causes of manic depression are still being researched in many areas including genetics, the immune system, viruses, brain biochemistry and structure, sleep and biorhythm disturbance, and hormones.

Genetics

As those of us who have relatives with mood disorders know, there's a strong hereditary element to manic depression. Greg has a pretty clear family history:

> There is no diagnosed history in my family, even though my father said in his generation and my generation there's been five suicides... There's a whole lot of undiagnosed bipolar running through both sides of my family... My grandmother was in Mont Park and I don't know if she was diagnosed as having Bipolar—this was probably in the late 60s, early 70s. Looking at her lifestyle, she had classic symptoms of bipolar. And she had a brother. We used to call him Uncle Tap—he either turned full on or turned full off. You couldn't shut him up, or you wouldn't see him for six months.

Jonathan, droll as ever, said: 'No one in my family had any evidence of manic depression except for my uncle, my father and my mother.'

Anita's mother, three uncles and two sons have had various, serious problems with moods. In fact, most people I spoke to could identify at least one family member who, if not formally diagnosed, suffered from significant mood disturbances. Sometimes a family history can be hidden. Mary said at first that she didn't have a family history of manic depression, but then:

I reckon my brother [who has alcoholic cirrhosis] could have it. Dad's sister had post-natal depression... And Dad said his cousin was, 'Never a happy man. Never a happy man. He had a car accident, but I know he killed himself.'

Genetic research has been going on for decades to try to isolate the gene or genes that are responsible. But scientists believe that the gene(s) that are linked with manic depression only create a *vulnerability to develop* the disorder. Once the vulnerability is there, all you need is a trigger event to kick the illness into action. (See Chapter 3.)

Immune system

Some scientists suspect that the immune system could be involved with manic depression. Blood levels of various elements of the immune system have been found to be significantly altered in people experiencing major depression. I have heard some people who take lithium for manic depression say proudly 'I never get a cold or the flu'. They tend to put themselves down as lucky. But there is some evidence that sufferers of asthma or hay fever (which are also associated with manic depression) have gained relief from lithium—but I wouldn't recommend taking it just to prevent a cold!

Some researchers[24] have suggested that an auto-immune phenomenon might be a clue to understanding the causes of manic depression. An auto-immune event is one in which the immune system turns on the body as if bits in the body were viruses. They cite, for example, the fact that people with multiple sclerosis, which is probably an auto-immune disease[25], have a much higher incidence of manic depressive symptoms than the rest of the population.[26]

Viruses

It is thought that viruses could cause manic depression. Mary had glandular fever at the age of nine. 'Not long after that,' she said, 'things started to go haywire—I started to have problems at school.' Jonathan said, 'I'd been a bit depressed and anorexic at school up 'til then, but in 1965 both Dad and I got a very bad flu, and that was when I had my first severe mood swings.'

The immune system's response to infection by a virus is to make an antibody. For each sort of virus, a specific sort of antibody is made. Once made, antibodies are like a cast made from the virus—antibody and virus match in a unique and specific way. Antibodies live on in the bloodstream after they've destroyed the virus. If a sample of your blood contains antibodies to virus A, then this is unmistakable evidence that you have come into contact with virus A.

Antibodies to the viruses that cause glandular fever, cold sores and some other conditions have been identified in the bloodstream of people with manic depression, whether or not they have had symptoms of those illnesses.[27] This raises the question as to whether these viruses could be causes of manic depression, but the research is still in its early days.

Brain biochemistry

Think of your brain as a robot's control system, jam-packed with electrical wires all linked up. In the brain, the wires are called nerve cells (neurons), and the connections are made not by solder, but by chemicals called neurotransmitters that 'swim' from one nerve cell to the next, passing on the 'current'.

Two of the neurotransmitters involved in manic depression are serotonin and dopamine. It is known that antidepressant medicines change the amount of neurotransmitters available to carry messages from one nerve cell to the next. Researchers hope that by discovering more about the way medicines work some light will be shed on the biochemical causes of manic depression.[28]

Structure of the brain

Studies of people who have diseases of the brain have suggested areas of the brain likely to be involved in creating symptoms of manic depression. Areas being researched include the systems controlled by the hypothalamus and pituitary gland (adrenal, thyroid and reproductive systems), the limbic system (emotional centre), the communication between the right and left hemispheres as well as parts of the cerebellum and the temporal lobe.

Much of this work is not directly relevant to living 'on the ground' with manic depression but it should continue to inform researchers and pharmacologists in the search for better diagnosis and treatments.

Sleep and biorhythm disturbance

Disturbance to sleep is a key *symptom* of most episodes of manic depression, but it is also likely that disturbance of sleep and the daily 'circadian' rhythms is a *cause* of manic depression.

There are a number of models about how this might work. One is the Sleep Deprivation Hypothesis which is based on the observation that sleep deprivation tends to elevate mood, both lifting depression and contributing to mania. It is thought that the loss of REM (Rapid Eye Movement) sleep—'dreaming sleep'—is responsible for this effect. Other factors thought to be causes of manic depression include the speed of the body clock and the sleep/wake cycle. The sleep/wake cycle is pushed ahead in depression.

Jonathan told me how this happened to him:

I have just recently had a terribly bad episode from September to June of not being able to sleep at all for up to three days... I would have been better off if I'd become nocturnal and slept in the daytime... but my psychiatrist wouldn't have that.

Hormonal factors

In women, hormones can be both a cause of manic depression and a trigger of episodes. It appears changes in reproductive hormones can directly cause severe and long-lasting episodes associated with events such as puberty, the menstrual cycle, pregnancy (including miscarriage and termination), childbirth and menopause.[29]

Other areas that could do with more investigation for both sexes are the adrenal and thyroid hormone systems which, along with reproductive hormones, are controlled by the same centres in the brain (hypothalamus and pituitary gland).

3

MAKING USE OF THE TECHNICAL STUFF

This chapter is about how we can make use of medical knowledge to start managing our own lives. We look at the inadequacy of the usual explanations of manic depression and consider another model; we discover the typical events that can trigger episodes; and how to use the information from Chapter 2 to get the message across to service providers.

THE MYTH OF THE WAVY LINE

According to most of the literature, Bipolar Disorder involves two separate states: mania and depression. The literature lists the symptoms, shows a wavy chart and implies that all we need to do to return to good health is to attend a psychiatrist and take lithium.

The first problem with this sort of simplistic explanation is that it denies the very common phenomenon of 'mixed states', where we can experience features of mania and depression at the same time. (See below for more information on mixed states.)

Another problem is that giving us lists of symptoms doesn't explain anything or help us manage our lives. Someone recovering from their first episode doesn't benefit by having their experiences minimised by being translated into jargon.

Finally, the wavy line implies that we're only 'normal' for a split second on the way up or down! What rot! The only

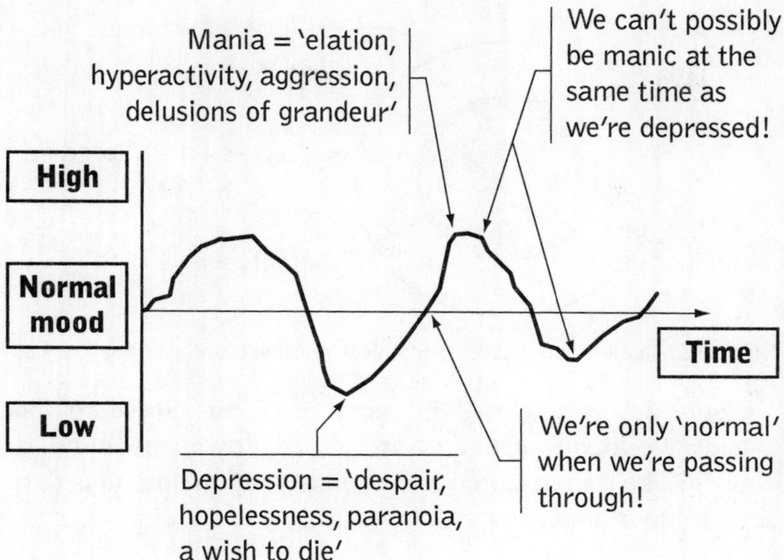

Figure 3.1 The 'wavy line' model of manic depression

useful thing about the wavy line is in illustrating how medicines work—see Chapter 4.

MORE ABOUT MOOD, ACTIVITY AND THINKING

A more useful model comes from the work of a psychiatrist named Kraepelin[1] who in 1921 observed that mood disorders affect three areas of life—mood, activity and thinking.

The white dots in Figure 3.2 represent where we're at in the range of mood, activity and thinking. The middle zone is the range of normal levels of mood, activity and thinking. The inner and outer zones represent the 'closed in' experience of depression and the 'blown out' experience of mania respectively.

In a 'pure' depressive state, mood, activity and thinking are all lowered. Winston Churchill called it his 'black dog'. I feel hopeless (mood), my thinking and concentration are sluggish (thinking) and I can't get out of bed (activity).

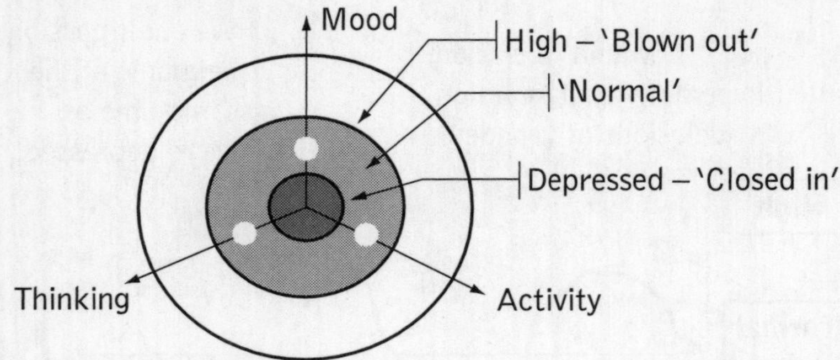

Figure 3.2 An alternative model for manic depression showing normal' range

Figure 3.3 is a 'closed in' situation: I am closed to the outside world, my activities are closed down, my mind is dimly lit like a shop closed for a holiday and my mood is flat, despairing or hopeless.

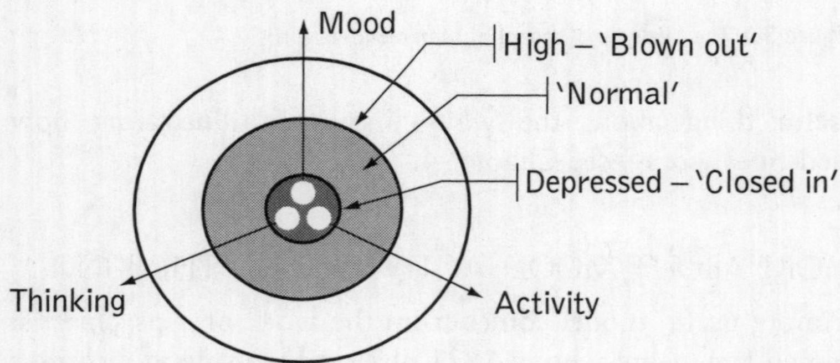

Figure 3.3 'Pure' depression

'Pure' mania, on the other hand, is utterly 'blown out'—I'm elated, feeling wonderful (mood); my thoughts are racing (thinking); I can't stop moving about or working or drinking (activity). Everything is exaggerated. (Figure 3.4)

Mixed states can also be drawn in this way. In 'black mania'[2] (depressive mania), I'm worried, depressed, and maybe paranoid. I'm constantly on the move, sleepless, very upset and compelled to resolve my worries immediately. (Figure 3.5)

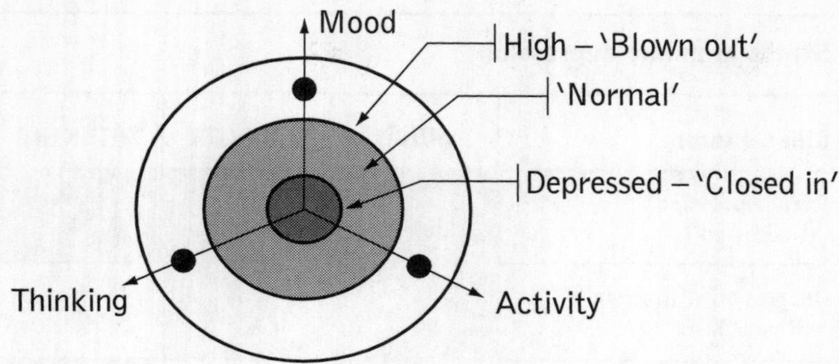

Figure 3.4 'Pure' mania

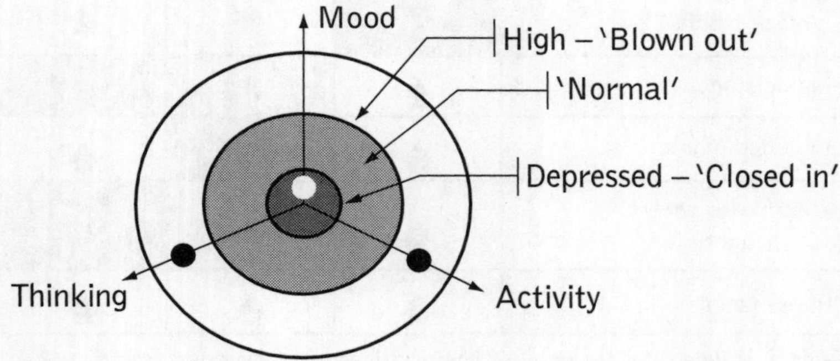

Figure 3.5 Black mania

Agitated depression is another mixed state. Here, depressed mood, stodgy thinking and 'suss' judgment combine with utter restlessness.

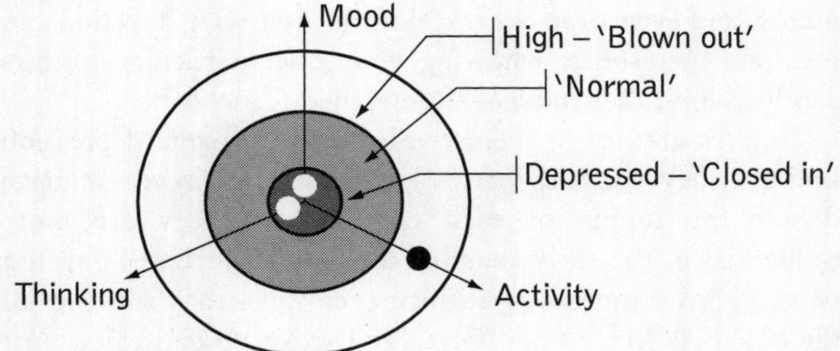

Figure 3.6 Agitated depression

States in manic depression			
Clinical term	**MOOD**	**ACTIVITY**	**THINKING**
Pure depression (black dog[3])	↓	↓	↓
Depression with flight of ideas	↓	↓	↑
Agitated depression	↓	↑	↓
Depressive mania (black mania[4])	↓	↑	↑
Manic stupor	↑	↓	↓
Inhibited mania	↑	↓	↑
Mania with poverty of thought	↑	↑	↓
Pure mania	↑	↑	↑

Table 3.1[5] illustrates the possible combinations of experiences.

TRIGGERS

Certain events can trigger episodes of mania and depression. Childbirth, other stressful life events, sleep loss, drugs, physical illness, and even overseas travel in the east-west direction can precipitate episodes. Knowing your own particular triggers can help limit the damage—forewarned is forearmed.

Triggers are not in themselves *causes* of manic depression nor are they episodes of it. Triggers do, however, tend to dictate the timing of each episode—and they are more influential in the early years of the condition. Later on, in a person who is not taking medicine, episodes may start out of the blue.[6] As Mary said: 'One day I woke up depressed. Just like that. Everything was fine...then overnight I felt shithouse.'

Reproductive events in women

Women with manic depression are at some risk of developing episodes at all key points in their reproductive lives including when they use oral contraceptives and hormone replacement therapy.[7]

Childbearing Childbirth is a potent trigger. Not only are there psychological stresses surrounding giving birth but there are also hormonal changes creating a whirlpool of changes in the mother,[8] and the associated sleep loss adds yet another trigger. Rachel has two children and has had a miscarriage and two abortions. Each pregnancy triggered a manic episode followed by depression.

Menstrual cycle Mood changes linked to the menstrual cycle have been known since Hippocrates and probably before. Understanding of the interaction between the menstrual cycle and exacerbated mood disturbance in women with manic depression has been poorly researched. However, things might be looking up with the inclusion of a new entity, 'Premenstrual Dysphoric Disorder' (PMDD) in DSM-IV. PMDD is severe and with more disturbing mood symptoms than the usual premenstrual syndrome (better known as PMT or premenstrual tension), and it affects around 3–8 per cent of women of reproductive age. The depressive symptoms of PMDD can sit on top of symptoms of one's manic depression, magnifying them so that it becomes difficult for the individual woman or her psychiatrist to determine just how well her manic depression is being controlled.[9]

The good news is that inclusion of PMDD in DSM-IV elevates the condition into a 'real' disorder—one which will probably attract more research, and more credibility among doctors.

Stress and trauma

Stressful life events can trigger episodes of manic depression. Grief and bereavement, changing jobs, divorcing or separating, moving house, and trauma such as bushfire, industrial accident, or being a victim of a crime can all act as triggers. Mara, a bank teller, had her mood disorder precipitated by an armed hold-up at work. She found her anxieties didn't improve over time as she expected, instead she was eventually hospitalised for depression. People who experienced abuse as children often link the abuse with the development of their mood disorder.

Biorhythms

Alterations to biorhythms through sleep disturbance, overseas travel and change in the seasons are thought to trigger manic depression.

Sleep disturbance Sleep loss is both a cause and a symptom of mania and it's probably the most-quoted warning sign of an imminent episode of mania. As Wendy said:

> The sleep is the key to the whole thing. If my sleep goes, it makes me more manic, and I'm tired from sleeplessness and I can't manage the mania as well.

Overseas travel There is some anecdotal evidence that east-west overseas travel can trigger mania. In other words, on a trip from Australia to Europe, you're better off travelling out through Los Angeles and coming home through Singapore.

Particular seasons

> *Melancholy occurs in autumn whereas mania in summer.*
>
> Posidonius, fourth century AD[10]

Posidonius' statement was rediscovered by twentieth century science. Mania does, indeed, occur mostly in summer. Further, there are two peak periods for major depression and suicide: autumn and spring. And, no surprise to those of us in the southern States, winter is a typical time to suffer depression, with its onset in April or May. In fact, the further towards the south pole you get, the more likely you are to suffer a winter depression. Researchers believe it is the number of hours of daylight that makes the difference.[11]

This reminds me of a friend whose psychiatrist had constructed for her a sort of permanent, portable summer for her to wear on her head. It consisted of a hard hat like those worn on construction sites. It had a short fluorescent tube fixed above the peak of the cap by bits of Meccano salvaged from some kid's bedroom floor. The light was carefully designed to simulate sunlight. My poor friend was bound by her word to wear this contraption day and night for as long as it took to see if it made any difference to her mood. Apparently the thing made no difference in the long run, but she did experience a lift in mood for a couple of days, not from the light contraption but from increased social interaction, as practically every patient, most nurses and some psychiatrists in the hospital stopped her, stifled their laughter and said 'What on earth is that on your head?'.

A seasonal predictability to one's mood shifts can be a blessing in disguise. If you know you're at risk at a certain time of the year you can take precautions: you might decide not to take holidays in July; you might decide, with your doctor, to start up antidepressants after Easter; and you will know to be careful to get regular hours of sleep in the lead-up to Christmas.

Drugs and alcohol

Some people can be tipped into hypomania by antidepressant medicines. Non-prescribed drugs and physical illness can also cause manic or depressive experiences, but this does not necessarily mean that the person has now developed manic depression.

Vince had used a number of recreational drugs for about a year and started to notice a link between feeling quite depressed and his use of these drugs. Fortunately when he stopped using the drugs, the fluctuating moods and depressions eased off.

Alcohol is a nervous system depressant. When we're depressed it's probably impossible to tell which part of our depression comes from having had too much to drink and which part of it is associated with manic depression. When my own depression lifted, however, I could definitely distinguish the jaded, tired form of 'depression' that alcohol causes from the lethargy of true melancholia.

Mind you, alcohol is used by many of us as a form of self-medication and paradoxically it can mask or disguise features of major depression or mania. As Marilyn observed, 'I was only diagnosed with manic depression after a skin complaint meant that I couldn't drink and my depression surfaced.'

Physical illness

A wide range of physical illnesses can act as a trigger for mood disturbance in three ways:

- the physical illness triggered an episode of manic depression (for example a viral illness); or
- the physical illness is directly causing symptoms that mimic manic depression (for example, AIDS dementia, some hormonal and metabolic conditions and cancers); or
- the treatment of the physical illness is interfering with treatment of manic depression (for example, a flare-up of a bowel problem limiting the amount of lithium that gets into the bloodstream).

GETTING THE MESSAGE ACROSS

Mary told me:

I was diagnosed as anorexic depressive and paranoid schizophrenic... I knew I wasn't anorexic ... I just didn't eat because I wasn't hungry ... They did those psychological tests on me...as a result of that they decided I was paranoid schizophrenic...I ended up in a private psychiatric hospital. I was only diagnosed with manic depression a couple of years after that.

Being wrongly diagnosed means missing out on the correct treatment and losing more years to manic depression. This was also Greg's experience:

It was the worst depression I'd ever had. I was totally withdrawn...I went back to my parents place...and I'd been there five, or seven days (I don't really know how long) without eating or drinking. That led to an almighty chase through the bush and I was carted off to Larundel...I was admitted to Larundel on Christmas Eve 1978...I was there for eight months and probably halfway through that I was on 1,800 milligrams of chlorprom Largactil® a day and still not sleeping. I went from...72 kilos down to something like 36 kilos.

I wasn't diagnosed as Bipolar until three years later... I was in hospital for six months, then this doctor put me on lithium and three weeks later I was out...

I reckon the best way for people to get diagnosed is to talk to other people within the ward.

I have to agree with Greg's last comment—only by learning, from whoever will tell us about our condition, can we tell psychiatrists about our experiences in a way they cannot misunderstand. If service providers cannot understand our language, we have to speak to them in theirs, or bear the consequences, as Angela's experience illustrates. A number of her close relatives have manic depression and the treating doctors knew of this, yet, as she told me:

When I was fifteen I got clinically depressed and I couldn't sleep and I was doing really silly things...I went to a GP. He gave me quite a bit of chlorprom which didn't touch me and so I went to hospital. I told them what I thought that I had manic depression but they treated me for schizophrenia because when they asked me if I heard voices in my head I said, 'Yes, we've all got a conscience.'

SO...NOW WHAT?

If you haven't been diagnosed with manic depression but you think you might have it, waste no more of your time and have an assessment through your general practitioner or a psychiatrist. If you're wrong, you'll be relieved. If you do have manic depression, the sooner you can take action, the sooner you will recover and get the most out of your life. The next chapter discusses what to expect from psychiatry.

4

WHAT'S ON OFFER FROM BIOLOGICAL PSYCHIATRY

In this chapter we'll explore the medicines and electroconvulsive therapy made available by 'biological' psychiatry, the branch of psychiatry that believes mental illness arises from biological, body-based changes to biochemistry and neuroanatomy.

TO TAKE OR NOT TO TAKE...

Although medicines and electroconvulsive therapy can relieve symptoms, achieving this isn't straightforward. First, most of us doubt the need for medicine or resist the idea of long-term medicine. Second, we have to discover which medicine suits us, is effective and doesn't give us unwanted side-effects.

Practically everyone tests the situation once by going off one or all of our prescribed drugs. Carole took herself off lithium and told me:

> I had felt well for a while and thought that would continue if I wasn't on medication ... I was well for about eighteen months and then I had a spot of depression ... Then I went on this almighty high...and ended up back in hospital.

After the high I got depressed so then I went back onto lithium.

Like most of us, Carole found herself learning the hard way:

During that time I had cancelled my health insurance because I thought that I was cured ... I had to pay back the hospital bill. I borrowed money from Dad.

After this episode, medicine was no longer an issue for Carole, even though it still presents hassles:

If you've got to go anywhere you've got to remember to have them [tablets] there. I find that a real drag because often I pack up and forget them. Last time that happened I was going away to Walhalla [Victoria] and I'd forgotten all my medication...I had to go to the chemist and beg for a strip of lithium. Fortunately I knew that chemist, and luckily I realised, because I was going away for three days ...

It's easy to forget, if you go out at night and come home and get into bed, lying there and remember: 'I haven't taken my tablets.' So then you lie there for another ten minutes cursing the fact that you haven't taken your tablets. Then eventually get up and begrudgingly swallow them. If I forget to take the [contraceptive] pill, that's one thing—but forgetting lithium could be life-threatening.

Kay Redfield Jamison, who co-authored the standard medical textbook *Manic-Depressive Illness*,[1] went on to become the Professor of Psychiatry at Johns Hopkins University and also happens to have manic depression, went off lithium and experienced disastrous consequences.

Even though I was a clinician and a scientist, and even though I could read the research literature and see the inevitable, bleak consequences of not taking lithium, I for many years after my initial diagnosis was reluctant to take my medications as prescribed ...Some of my reluctance stemmed from a fundamental denial that I had a disease...and it was difficult to give up the high flights of mind and mood, even though the depressions that inevitably followed nearly cost me my life.[2]

Almost all of us want to believe that our manic depression is something we can beat on our own, without medicine and without a label. It's a natural human reaction to the notion of madness to try to prove to ourselves and those around us that we were never mad in the first place, or if we were, it was a 'one-off' that doesn't mean we're destined for more madness.[3]

People around us can influence our decision to stop taking medicines. Anita told me: 'I went off it, and had three close friends telling me I didn't need it, and that there's nothing wrong with me. So I didn't see my doctor, who ended up putting me in hospital again.'

And Carole: 'My in-laws held a lot of resentment...they were really against my taking medication. They felt I could get better just by trying to help myself a bit more.'

If you do go off your medicine, don't be ashamed—you will have learned a great deal from your own experience and you'll be in a better position to make your own decision about treatment.

Medicine for manic depression comes in three main groups:

- mood stabilisers;
- mood lifters; and
- 'symptom settlers'.

Each of these works on one or more of mood, activity and thinking.

MOOD STABILISERS

Mood stabilisers work on each of mood, activity and thinking, bringing each factor back towards the normal range. They have varying degrees of 'antimanic' and 'antidepressant'

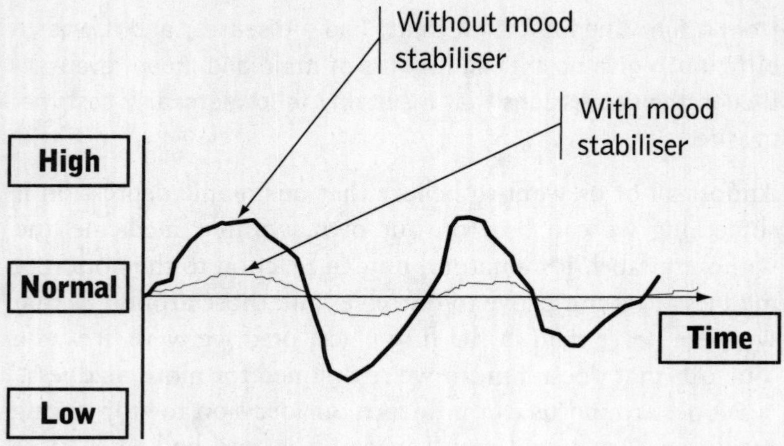

Figure 4.1 Action of mood stabilisers

action. The 'wavy line' graph illustrates their action on mood, flattening out the peaks and troughs.

The mood stabilisers currently in use in Australia are lithium carbonate (Lithicarb® and Quilonum-SR®) and three drugs from the anticonvulsant (anti-epileptic) group.

Lithium

Lithium was discovered to relieve mania in 1948 by the Australian psychiatrist Dr John Cade.[4] However, it wasn't until the early 1970s that people with manic depression began to be treated with lithium and it became the main treatment for manic depression.

Lithium is most effective for people with Bipolar I or II and less so with Major Depressive Disorder. Lithium is both an antimanic and an antidepressant medicine. Its antidepressant action is more effective for people with Bipolar illness than those with Major Depressive Disorder.[5] Because of this, antidepressant medicine is often given as well as lithium, in which case the lithium adds to the effect of the antidepressant.[6]

Lithium has some effect in 80–90 per cent of people with manic depression,[7] but only 75 per cent of people taking lithium will be relieved of major mood shifts altogether.[8] Lithium's beneficial effects can start modestly and increase for up to twelve months before the full benefit is gained.

Lithium can be used by most people, but if you have heart failure, kidney or thyroid problems or Addison's disease you should only be given lithium as a last resort and only after you have discussed all the risks with your doctor (and preferably obtained a second, independent opinion) as lithium can exacerbate these conditions. Lithium causes birth defects (mainly heart abnormalities) in around 10 per cent of pregnancies. Unwanted effects of lithium are shown in Table 4.1.

To be effective, lithium needs to be taken at a high dose—close to the toxic level. This is why regular blood lithium levels should be taken so that the daily dose can be altered to keep the blood level in the safe, effective range of 0.8–1.6 mmol/L.

You can become toxic if the daily dose is too high, you've taken an overdose or if the weather is hot, especially if you become dehydrated at any time. The signs of toxicity include loss of appetite, nausea, vomiting, abdominal pain, diarrhoea, staggering, slurred speech, marked tremor and agitation.

Lithium toxicity is dangerous. If you do become toxic, immediately:

- stop taking lithium;
- drink at least one litre of fluid per hour; and
- contact your doctor or go to a hospital.[13]

Anticonvulsants

This class of drug is a double act—first developed for their effectiveness in controlling the seizures of epilepsy, they also act as mood stabilisers. Anticonvulsants used for manic depression in Australia are carbamazepine (Tegretol®), sodium valproate (Epilim®) and clonazepam (Rivotril®).

A number of people who'd been on lithium have told me that switching to anticonvulsants gave them, within two or three days, a more tangible calmness and stability of mood

Unwanted effects of lithium	Solutions
Memory loss and impaired or slowed thinking[9]	None effective. Try carrying a notebook and remember to refer to it.
Weight gain[10]	Don't drink soft drink or juice to slake your thirst.
Muscular unco-ordination, especially noticeable when playing sport;[11] tremor.	None effective. Some people can change their golf or tennis swing; others take up less demanding sporting styles.
Sense of flatness	May be dose-related, or unaccustomed 'stability' of mood. Speak to prescribing doctor to see about reducing the dose.
Blunted creativity[12]	None effective.
Acne, dry skin	Seek advice from a general practitioner.
Nausea, vomiting, diarrhoea	Take lithium on full stomach, with milk. Try a 'slow-release' lithium preparation if available.
Thirst	This is because lithium is a salt. Carry a bottle of water with you. Limit alcohol intake as the dehydrating effect of alcohol is increased by lithium.
Thyroid problems	A blood test should be carried out every year so any thyroid problem can be identified, before any serious or irreparable damage is done. Treatment with thyroid hormone if necessary.
Passing lots of urine	Caused by kidneys being affected by the lithium and not concentrating urine as they used to, and/or by drinking more because you're thirsty. A kidney function test should be done every year to check there is no permanent damage being done to the kidneys.

Table 4.1 Unwanted effects of lithium

than they'd experienced on lithium. On the other hand many people suffer terribly from unwanted effects.

Unwanted effects may be dose related—in other words, starting when the dose is increased and disappearing when lowered. Other effects might be a major nuisance when you first start the medicine but eventually disappear over a period of time. Or you might find they don't let up. If they're causing too much of a problem you might need to come off the medicine.

Keep the patient information sheet that comes with the pack and if you have any unwanted effect or other health problem develop while on anticonvulsant medicine, discuss it with your psychiatrist.

Carbamazepine and valproate Unwanted effects are too numerous to list fully here, but include nausea, vomiting, headache, drowsiness, double vision, confusion, blood and liver disorders. The toxic effects are exaggerations of the unwanted effects and can include respiratory failure, coma and death.

If you are pregnant, or have glaucoma, liver disorder, diabetes, a blood disorder or kidney problems, you should discuss the fact with your doctor.

Carbamazepine can decrease the effectiveness of the oral contraceptive Pill and cause 'breakthrough' bleeding throughout the month.

Clonazepam Clonazepam, a drug from the benzodiazepine (for example Valium®) class, has a different set of unwanted effects including sedation, 'behaviour problems', fatigue and muscle weakness. Toxic and overdose effects include exaggerations of the unwanted effects and respiratory and heart problems.

MOOD LIFTERS

Mood lifters (antidepressants) act on mood, activity and thinking to bring each factor back to normal from the 'closed in' range, as shown in Figure 4.2. The wavy line illustrates their action on mood by simply lifting the troughs 'upwards'. We'll have a look at the three main groups—older 'tricyclic' and 'MAOI' antidepressants, and the newer 'serotonin' ones.

Tricyclic and tetracyclic antidepressants

These get their name from the number of 'benzene rings' in their chemical structures. Some of the brands on the market in Australia are listed in Table 4.3.

These medicines can take a couple of weeks before they have an effect on mood, so you have to be prepared to be patient.

Unwanted effects can be a problem. These older drugs act on the brain not only to lessen depression, but they also affect other body systems. Because this group has similar chemical structure and actions, the unwanted effects tend to be similar. The following reactions affect most people: dry mouth, constipation, blurred vision, weight gain, drowsiness and dizziness or fainting. A wide range of less common effects can also occur. Check these on the patient information sheet in the pack or ask your doctor.

Medicines in this class are not addictive but if you stop them suddenly you might feel 'off colour', nauseated, or get headaches, so it's best to reduce the dose gradually over a week or two.

An overdose of tricyclics will principally attack the heart, causing irregularities in the heart beat, a drop in blood pressure and heart attack. Overdosage can also cause confusion, hallucinations, agitation, vomiting, coma and death. Treatment for overdose involves emptying the stomach by pumping or charcoal, then attention to preventing death from heart attack. Overdose of tetracyclics can cause confusion, drowsiness, convulsions and coma.

If you have prostate problems, heart disease, epilepsy, hyperthyroidism or glaucoma, tell your doctor as tricyclics must be used with caution when these conditions are present.

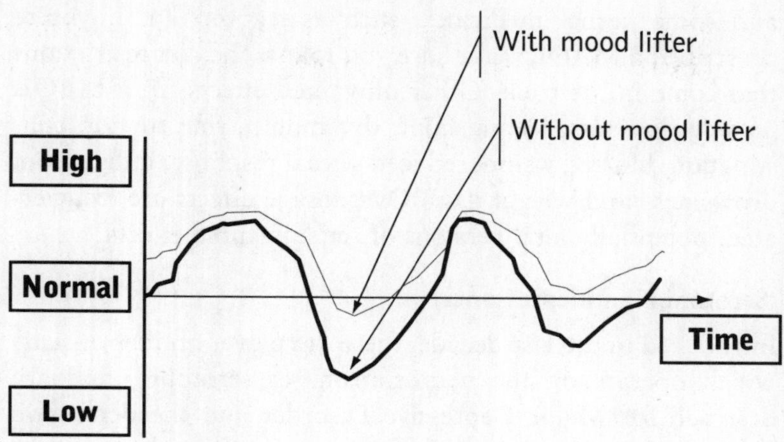

Figure 4.2 Action of mood lifters

It is not recommended that women use tricyclics during pregnancy or breastfeeding as tricyclics rarely cause damage to the foetus and are excreted in breast milk. Certain exceptions may be made to this rule of thumb depending on your overall situation.

Monoamine oxidase inhibitors (MAOIs)

Usually pronounced 'mayos' these drugs include tranylcypromine (Parnate®) and phenelzine (Nardil®). MAOIs are stronger than tricyclics, but are less often used now because of the risks of high blood pressure and stroke, and the necessary dietary restrictions (see below).

Let your doctor know, and discuss with him/her the pros and cons of taking MAOIs if you have diabetes, epilepsy or a condition affecting the liver, kidney, heart or thyroid. MAOIs should be avoided if possible during pregnancy.

MAOIs will cause a sudden, steep rise in blood pressure if you have tyramine in your diet. The rise in blood pressure can lead to stroke. This means a longish list of forbidden foods, such as cheese, more than three glasses of wine, Vegemite®, and some herbal medicines, such as tryptophan. If you're prescribed a MAOI, make sure you follow the diet restrictions that come in the pack. Other unwanted effects from MAOIs include dizziness, feeling faint, dry mouth, fine tremor, constipation, blurred vision, reduced sexual response, indigestion, drowsiness and weight gain. Overdosage effects are exaggerated, potentially fatal versions of the unwanted effects.

'Serotonin' antidepressants

Introduced in the last decade, these are newer antidepressants which operate on the neurotransmitter serotonin, and are designed for Major Depressive Disorder and the depressive phase of Bipolar illness. They are more effective, can take effect in as little as a couple of days and, unlike older antidepressants, it's less likely you'll get unwanted effects—you probably won't know you're on them. Brands available in Australia include sertraline (Zoloft®), fluoxetine (for example, Prozac®), paroxetine (Aropax20®), venlafaxine (Efexor®), nefazodone (Serzone®) and citalopram (Cipramil®).

If you have a condition affecting your heart, kidneys, liver or if you have epilepsy, discuss it with your prescribing doctor. Prozac® attracted a bad name after it was alleged that aggressive behaviour was an unwanted effect, albeit rare.[14]

The 'serotonin antidepressants' can all activate mania or hypomania, and they can all ruin your sex life. As well, each can cause a number of different unwanted effects. With new drugs, knowledge about the range of unwanted effects is limited, so discuss any unexpected medical event with your psychiatrist and check the patient information sheet.

An overdose on these drugs causes nausea, vomiting, agitation, restlessness and hypomania. They are claimed, based on the limited information available at this stage, to have a wide 'safety margin' when taken alone (that is, not combined with alcohol or other medicines).

'SYMPTOM SETTLERS'

Alcohol, marijuana and opium have been used to quieten extremes of distress since time immemorial, but the first Western psychiatric drugs only became available in the 1950s.

Drugs in this category include antipsychotics and benzodiazepines. They have little or no effect on mood, but can settle disturbed 'blown out' levels of activity and thinking.

Antipsychotic agents

Chlorpromazine (Largactil®), thioridazine (Melleril®), trifluoperazine (Stelazine®) and haloperidol (Serenace®) are examples of antipsychotics that have been traditionally used in Australia. These are older drugs, widely critised for their capacity to cause sedation (the feeling of trying to swim through peanut butter or trying to make a decision in a dream) and because they have serious and potentially life-threatening effects.

In the last decade newer 'atypical' antipsychotics were developed for people with schizophrenia and two of these—risperidone (Risperdal®) and olanzapine (Zyprexa®)—may be used in Australia for the treatment of severe acute manic depression. These drugs appear to be more effective in controlling symptoms and are claimed to be 'safer', but they still carry serious risks.

However, the antipsychotics most commonly used in Australia these days are still the older and cheaper ones.[15] Some leading psychiatrists are now privately calling for a change in prescribing habits, saying older antipsychotics are 'making people sicker', and they are used for too long (that is, they are continued after the crisis of the episode has passed).[16] Less damaging options suggested for people suffering severe acute mania include treatment with 'atypical' antipsychotics or another group of drugs altogether—benzodiazepines (see below).

If your psychiatrist suggests you take an antipsychotic medicine, he or she should ask if you have epilepsy, kidney problems, liver problems, problems with your white blood cells or if you're pregnant. Discuss the risks before you agree to take antipsychotics (that is, if you're allowed to consent).

Unwanted effects vary according to the particular medicine and the next best source of information after your psychiatrist is the patient information sheet that should come with the medicine. If you don't get that information, ask other people who are also using the same or similar medicines. If you experience anything out of the ordinary while taking these medicines, let your doctor know.

Risks from all antipsychotic medicines All antipsychotic drugs can cause weight gain and sedation. In addition, there are two damaging effects that are rare but you should know about: tardive dyskinesia and neuroleptic malignant syndrome. The newer 'atypical' antipsychotics are claimed to be less likely to cause tardive dyskinesia and neuroleptic syndrome but the cautions still apply.[17, 18]

TARDIVE DYSKINESIA Tardive dyskinesia involves involuntary twitchiness and rhythmic movements such as chewing movements in the muscles of your face and mouth. No one quite knows how the drugs cause it and there is no effective treatment.[19]

The best bet is to talk with a trusted doctor about it and see if there are any realistic options to reduce your risk.

NEUROLEPTIC MALIGNANT SYNDROME Neuroleptic malignant syndrome is a potentially fatal but rare condition in which you get rigid muscles, fever, sweating, difficulty breathing and confusion. If this happens, get to the nearest public hospital as fast as you can.

Benzodiazepines

One of the benzodiazepines, clonazepam, mentioned above as a 'mood stabliser' is also a 'symptom settler'. Clonazepam has also been shown by some studies[20] to be as effective in treating acute mania as older antipsychotics. Unwanted effects of clonazepam have been discussed above. Like other benzodiazepines, clonazepam causes dependence and abrupt withdrawal may cause a sudden re-emergence of symptoms.[21]

Medicines and childbearing

Lithium *can* be used in pregnancy but generally not in the first trimester, as the baby would run a 5–10 per cent risk of having heart or other abnormalities. Being on lithium doesn't necessarily mean you can't have children. If you take lithium and fall pregnant or are planning a pregnancy, talk to your doctor sooner rather than later.

Very little information about the use of 'serotonin antidepressants' in pregnancy has been gathered. The prescribing notes provided by the manufacturers say '... this drug should be used in pregnancy only if clearly needed'.

It is possible to manage a pregnancy and childbearing stage whilst on medicine for a mood disorder but it takes commitment, perhaps a little creativity and certainly a lot of discussion between you, your partner and your doctor to achieve it. It might involve running the 13 weeks' gauntlet during the first trimester without any psychiatric drugs and then progressively reintroducing them; it might mean some other rearrangement of medicine, or adding healing from an advanced chiropractor or reiki practitioner—either way, and despite the warnings listed above, there's not necessarily any reason why your manic depression should automatically mean childbearing is out of the question. Some of the other issues involved in making decisions about childbearing are discussed in Chapter 13.

Weight gain

Many people experience unwanted weight gain while being treated with psychiatric medicines, particularly when treatment is prolonged or indefinite. Although factors such as lower levels

Type of medicine	Sub-type	Brand name (example)	Generic name	What it does
Mood stabilisers	Anticonvulsant	Tegretol® Epilim® Rivotril®	carbamazepine sodium valproate clonazepam	Limits the extent of the mood shift
	Lithium carbonate	Lithicarb® Quilonum–SR®	lithium carbonate	Limits the extent of the mood shift
Mood lifters	'Serotonin' antidepressants	Zoloft® Prozac® Aropax 20® Efexor® Serzone® Cipramil®	sertraline fluoxetine paroxetine venlafaxine sertraline citalopram	Lifts the mood
	Tricyclics	Prothiaden® Tofranil® Tryptanol® Sinequan® Anafranil® Surmontil®	dothiepin imiprimine amitriptyline doxepin clomipramine trimipramine	Lifts the mood

Table 4.3 Some of the medicines commonly prescribed for manic depression in Australia and their uses

Type of medicine	Sub-type	Brand name (example)	Generic name	What it does
	Tetracyclic	Tolvon®	mianserin	Lifts the mood
	Others	Aurorix®	moclobemide	Lifts the mood
	MAOIs	Nardil® Parnate®	phenelzine tranylcypromine	Lifts the mood
Symptom settlers	Antipsychotics (older)	Melleril® Largactil® Stelazine® Serenace®	thioridazine chlorpromazine trifluoperazine haloperidol	Settles the hyperactivity and racing thoughts of mania
	Antipsychotics (atypical, newer)	Risperdal® Zyprexa®	risperidone olanzapine	As above
	Benzodiazepines	Rivotril®	clonazepam	As above

Table 4.3 (cont) Some of the medicines commonly prescribed for manic depression in Australia and their uses

of physical activity associated with being ill can contribute, it is accepted that some medicines do cause weight gain.[22] Ask your psychiatrist to weigh you regularly during treatment and when you start on a new medicine. You can also ask to see a dietitian at your community or mental health clinic.

ELECTROCONVULSIVE (SHOCK) TREATMENT

It has been established that electroconvulsive therapy (ECT) can offer a fast solution to the severest depression, even when antidepressants have failed. ECT is probably the single most feared aspect of the practice of psychiatry. In 1941, when ECT was introduced in Australia, the practice was relatively barbaric. Two electrodes were placed on the temples and an electric shock was sent through the electrodes to the individual. The patient would undergo a convulsion not unlike an epileptic seizure, requiring six or so hospital staff to hold the convulsing patient to prevent the convulsion from causing injuries. In the 1990s ECT is administered after an injection of a muscle relaxant (Scoline®) and a general anaesthetic, so there are no screams, no convulsion and minimal risk of physical injury.

Everyone has an opinion on electroconvulsive therapy (ECT), including those who know nothing of the procedure or nothing of mental illness. For example, in 1976, during the construction of Australia's largest psychiatric centre, the architect wouldn't believe the psychiatrist briefing him that sound-proofing in the ECT room was unnecessary—he'd seen *One Flew Over the Cuckoo's Nest*—and went ahead and put lead in the wall anyway.[23]

When I had ECT, I had elliptical pink marks from the electrodes at both temples for some time after the treatment. I could function minute by minute but I couldn't resume living alone for several months. I'll never know how much of that was caused by the depression (which hadn't lifted) or the ECT. Carole's experience was similar, having had ECT: 'Once, about fifteen years ago (and it didn't really help) and again about eighteen months ago (and it didn't really help.)'

Others, like Mary, who said 'Next time I get depressed, no mucking around. I'm having ECT straight away—it works so fast', and Jonathan are pragmatic. Jonathan's doctor recommended ECT after his condition deteriorated in hospital.

> He explained ECT to me and my parents as a sledgehammer technique which they use to save time because it was just impossible for them to get someone to watch me 24 hours a day. If I was going to suicide, I would do it some way. And ECT would bring me out of a suicidal and critical state more quickly ... I was booked for six sessions ... They gave me injections to knock me out at about a quarter past eight in the morning, and at a quarter past nine I'd be woken up by the nurse bringing breakfast in. I felt quite well ... My writing had deteriorated by that stage ... because I had the shakes. After the first session of ECT it was amazing to see my writing straighten up, straight away. After two sessions, my doctor said I didn't need any more because I'd responded so well...

The Burdekin inquiry found 'most consumers expressed a deep personal fear and rejection of ECT yet most psychiatrists who mentioned it viewed it simply as a "treatment option"'.[24] ECT is used most commonly for depression, but also in some cases for mania.

We have the right to consent to having ECT. However, it can be difficult to withhold consent because mental health laws allow psychiatrists to override our refusal in certain circumstances if we are 'unable' to consent or decline to consent. See Appendix III for avenues of assistance with rights.

How does ECT work?

The details of how ECT works are not known for sure. ECT, like many psychiatric medicines, was discovered by chance to influence depression.[25] Only after that observation was its mechanism of action studied. It is known that the seizure itself, rather than the electric current, causes the individual's response to ECT. Researchers are now studying the effects of ECT on a wide range of neurotransmitters.[26]

Risks—are they real and do they matter?

The risks appear to be primarily from the anaesthetic. As with any procedure involving a general anaesthetic, there is some risk. As for the unwanted effects of ECT itself, the answer you get depends on whom you talk to. Some researchers claim there is no risk. Others admit that it causes memory loss and disruption to other thinking processes but suggest it is temporary and reversible. Others suggest permanent damage takes place. It appears that factors such as whether one or two electrodes are used, the amount of the electric charge and the duration of the charge could influence the degree of brain damage.

Some undisputed facts about ECT

- When it works, ECT lifts depression.
- When it works, ECT works fast.
- ECT happens under general anaesthetic and with a muscle relaxant and there are no convulsions or screams.
- ECT has temporary unwanted effects on memory and other brain functions.

WEIGHING UP THE RISKS — A TWENTIETH CENTURY LUXURY

I will say nothing against the course of my existence. But at bottom it has been nothing but pain and burden, and I can affirm that during the whole of my 75 years, I have not had four weeks of genuine well-being. It is but the perpetual rolling of a rock that must be raised up again forever.

Goethe[27]

Johann Wolfgang von Goethe, Napoleon Bonaparte, William Blake, Theodore Roosevelt, Oliver Cromwell, Virginia Woolf and a host of other notable people made a significant contribution in their fields despite a lifetime battling manic depression without any of the psychiatric treatment we have available today.

In the latter half of the twentieth century there was a proliferation of treatments for manic depression. These days we have choices (unless the law forces our hand—see Chapter 7). Notionally, we are now able to choose whether to use psychiatric medicine to relieve the pain of manic depression, or go with our own rhythms and thereby reap the many benefits of the insights, achievements and experiences born of ecstasy, despair, creativity and drive.

My years at medical school and the conservatism the course taught me are often at odds with my own experience of chronic illness. That conservatism and 'common sense' approach would have us accept without question the 'need' for permanent preventative treatment.

But I, like many others, have had to weigh up the pros and cons. For example, if I want my mind to work at its best, or if I want to enjoy my sexuality to the full, I can choose to go without certain medicines, running the risk of becoming ill again. On the other hand, I tell myself, I *don't* have to suffer intolerable pain—all I have to do is to get onto the medicine and run the risk of suffering its short- or long-term damage.

Get as much information as you can and make a choice. If the choice involves weighing up risks, then only you can choose among the risks. Sometimes you have to settle for the 'least worst' option, but always remember you don't have to suffer intolerable pain or distress.

5

TALKING AND ALTERNATIVE THERAPIES

TALKING THERAPIES

The term 'talking therapies' covers a wide range of activities—from the confessional to getting advice from a friend, from rational thinking to dynamic psychotherapy, from family therapy to problem-solving counselling.

Cognitive behavioural therapy

The words 'cognitive', 'cognisance', 'recognise' etc. all come from the Latin root, *cognoscere*, to get to know or investigate. For practical purposes, cognitive therapy relies on getting us to get to know how our thinking influences our feelings—there are ways of thinking that prolong distress and ways of thinking that limit it.

Intuitively, we know that mood, activity and thinking all influence each other.

We're all too aware of mood acting on activity, for example, we stay under the doona, or we don't pick up the phone. However, it also works the other way around: if I'm depressed and I force myself to do some painting, or running, or whatever, my mood starts to improve, a little, if only temporarily.

We can see our thoughts influencing activity every time we make a decision. I've found that the reverse is also true: my activities do change my thinking. For example, after a stressful day, taking my dog for a walk helps me to relax and to stop thinking about the day's issues.

We know, too, how mood acts on thinking. In an elated mood, I know I can do the Prime Minister's job at the same time as negotiating permanent peace in Northern Ireland and the Middle East; but when I'm depressed, I think I'm worthless, that I'll never be out of the abyss. Our mood affects our thinking, but can our thinking affect our mood? Cognitive behavourial therapy, for example Albert Ellis' version called Rational Emotive Therapy[1] believes so.

RATIONAL EMOTIVE THERAPY (RET) Albert Ellis' theories are simple and easy to remember. He points out that most people consider that their feelings are *directly created* by events in their lives.

However, Ellis reasons that in between the activating event and our consequential feelings, there are our *beliefs*. His A, B, C of rational thinking are overleaf.

THREE FUNDAMENTAL IRRATIONAL BELIEFS Ellis identified three basic irrational beliefs[2] that we commonly use with destructive consequences. These beliefs are relevant to living with manic depression.

1. 'I must do well and win approval or else I am an inadequate, rotten person.' (For example, 'I must never be depressed because that doesn't meet with others' approval and if I do get depressed, it's because I'm inadequate and too needy.')

2. 'Others must treat me considerately and kindly in precisely the way I want them to treat me; if they don't, society and the universe should severely blame, damn and punish them for their inconsiderateness.' (For example, 'My family should not have called the crisis team and insisted that I go to hospital, because I'm not sick and don't want to be labelled or locked up. It's their fault I'm in hospital and they should be punished.')

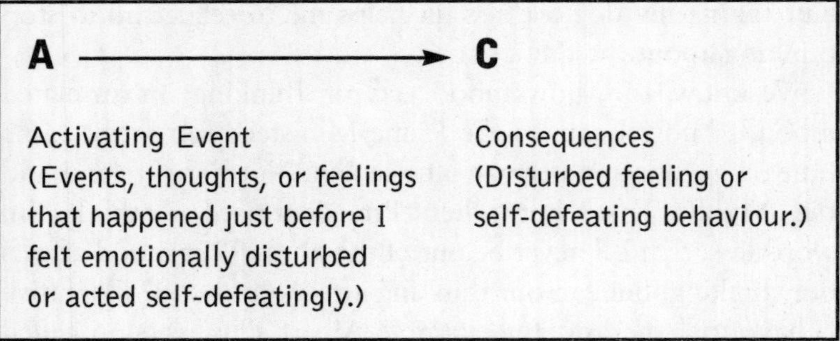

Table 5.1 The popular misconception. Adapted from Bernard, 1986[3]

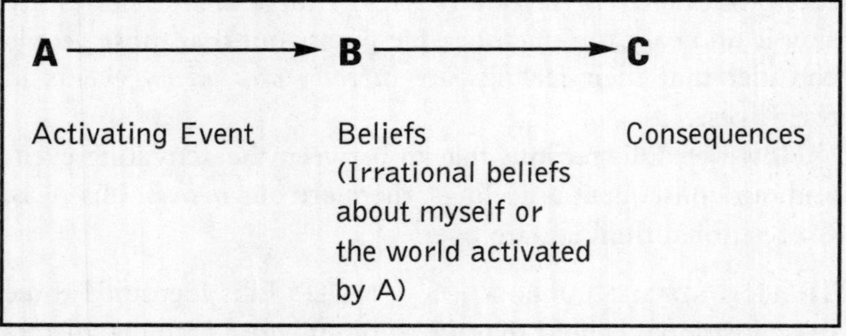

Table 5.2 How irrational beliefs, not events, cause disturbed feelings and self-defeating behaviour. Adapted from Bernard, 1986[4]

3. 'Conditions under which I live must be arranged so that I get practically everything I want comfortably, quickly and easily, and receive nothing that I don't want.' (For example, 'I should not have gotten manic depression because it's not fair and I don't deserve it.')

RET points out that by using the concepts of 'must' and 'should' we turn wishful thinking into something we can only be angry and upset about. If we try to insist that other people and the universe should be anything better than they are, we're ignoring logic. Why *must* we be treated well? Why *must* life turn out exactly as we want? There's no universal law that says so. In fact, the evidence that the world is full of undesirable events is in our faces every day in the news.

Here is an example relevant to life on the roller-coaster.

A — Activating event	B — Beliefs	C — Consequences	D — Dispute	E — Effective beliefs
Doctor puts me off work for three months	My boss will definitely sack me when I try to return.	I feel angry and rejected.	Where is the law that says my boss will sack me?	So what if he finds out? There are laws to stop him from sacking me just because I've been ill.
	I'll never be well enough to go back to work.	I get more depressed and my self-esteem plummets.	Three months is not 'never'. Keep specific and don't 'awfulise'.	I'd prefer to continue on at work but I can't at the moment. This illness comes and goes and I will recover from this episode.
	I won't have enough money to pay the rent and I'll be forced onto the streets.	I panic and get really angry.	I don't deserve anything, good or bad. I can choose to be homeless or borrow money for rent or move to a cheaper place.	I don't like having to move, or borrow money or even rely on shelters, but I won't starve.

Table 5.4 Example of using Ellis' system for life on the roller-coaster

Ellis advises us that we would be better off if we stopped insisting that the world be as we wished it and accepted that the world and the people in it are not answerable to us. Then we can start turning the irrational beliefs into useful positions. For example:

1. 'It would be nice to be approved of 100 per cent of the time by others but they don't have to. If my depression upsets my family, I can try to do something about that but their upset doesn't mean I'm inadequate.'
2. 'It would be better if the situation hadn't turned out that my family had me admitted to hospital, but they did. There's no law that says my family always have to do what I want. I'm in here now and I'd better not waste energy getting upset about something that's already happened.'
3. 'It would have suited me much better not to have gotten manic depression. It isn't fair and I don't deserve it but there's no guarantee that the universe will protect me from unfairness.'

THE 'TYRANNY OF THE SHOULDS'[5] The idea that unifies these irrational beliefs is that we turn rational *preferences* into irrational *should* or *must* statements.[6] 'Should' is Albert Ellis' dirty word. A six-letter word that ought to be spelled IT-WOULD-BE-BETTER-IF. It sounds strange, but try introducing a ban on the word 'should' in your household (permit 'it would be better if…') and after a month see if the household isn't functioning more smoothly.

AWFULISING Hand in hand with the 'shoulds', the widespread practice of 'awfulising' makes us feel even worse. Ellis prompts us to answer honestly the question, 'What is the absolute worst thing that can happen?' Using our three examples we can see where 'awfulising' creeps in.

1. 'It's absolutely awful and I can't stand it when my family blames me for upsetting them when I'm depressed. My family's acceptance is so important to me that I can't live without it.'
2. 'It's the end of my life as I know it now I've come into a mental hospital. Now everyone will call me crazy and I'll be crazy for life. I might as well give up now. My family really has a lot to answer for, wrecking my life like this.'
3. 'Manic depression means I'll never hold down a job, my partner will probably leave me and I'll never be able to achieve what I wanted to achieve.'

We can use logical counter-arguments to awfulising in the same way as we beat the 'shoulds'. For example, after 'de-awfulising' the statements above, they could become:

1. 'I'd strongly prefer it if my family didn't get so upset when I'm depressed. But that's not the worst thing that could possibly happen to me. Even if my partner and children left, I would still be able to survive.'
2. 'Some people might treat me badly because I've been in a mental hospital but not everyone. If people treat me badly, that's not the end of the world.'
3. 'Manic depression might cause problems with my job and my partner and I might have to make other plans but even if that happened it wouldn't kill me.'

UPSETTING OURSELVES BECAUSE WE'RE UPSET Ellis also observed that people get upset because they're insisting to themselves that they shouldn't feel a particular way—angry, confused, incompetent, too happy.[7] Getting cross or upset because manic depression has returned can lead us to panic and make things worse for ourselves.

A reflection on RET

For about eight years I lived on conning myself...I came up with all these motivational sayings...and just living on a belief that I really didn't believe in, but I had nothing else solid to grab hold of. So I made this fake belief thing so I could hang onto that, hoping that it would be a way to get through—and it was! It became real when I started achieving stuff.

Paul

On the eve of my dismissal from hospital, where I'd spent six weeks in intensive, nine-to-five group and one-to-one work on cognitive techniques, I suddenly realised that I was still profoundly depressed. I just 'knew' that the new way of thinking I'd been taught was false, inconsistent with my experience and that I would be kidding myself if I thought I was worthy of more than the lifted hind leg of a dog. The nurse was empathetic but she would not budge: cognitive techniques did work; in fact it was the only means she knew of by which to beat depression.

Those of us who've been bothered by severe, recurring depression have met this approach before in the pages of thousands of paperbacks in the 'psychology/self help' section at the bookshop. I've read them all over the last twenty years (or it seems like it). They all peddle the same wares: We are responsible for our emotional responses. We can change our emotional responses with our thoughts.

The problem is that in the grip of a depressive episode our capacity to choose between two different ways of thinking is severely limited. Our thoughts are abysmally negative, irrational—we are convinced of our own shame, guilt, worthlessness. It is therefore impossible for us to faithfully adopt a belief of our worthiness. If we do adopt this belief, it inevitably feels like a false belief. It can even become a 'should' in its own right—'I should try harder to believe that cognitive techniques are useful!' I came to believe that the failure couldn't come from the techniques I was taught, so it must be me who was to blame for the lack of relief from my symptoms.

To my surprise, I found that adopting this 'false belief' against my better judgment was useful in the long run, but only when the medicine had started to lift the worst of the depression.

As my mood lifted, I realised that I was now starting to use clear thinking techniques to prevent my mood diving in response to either the thoughts of my daydreams or the thousand little situations of daily life. I realised that cognitive techniques can keep reactive depression at bay and keep me going in the face of both hypomania and depression. Since then I've come to the conclusion that Rational Emotive Therapy works, but to give it its best chance remember:

a. not much lasting change happens unless your mood state is relatively stable. While we are ill, we can't comprehend new information as well as usual, and our ability to see the value of this approach is limited; and

b. to make effective changes you need time, effective healing and determination.

One final point: cognitive behavioural therapy leaves little room for spiritual belief. Albert Ellis passes religion off as either 'strong philosophy' or a 'faith unfounded in fact, in dogma, absolutistic thinking…there is one God [who] tells us what you *should* do.'[8] This is discussed further in Chapter 14.

Psychotherapy

Pronounced 'sick o'therapy' by my child, this is a mixed bag of techniques and theories. Some particular types include:

- psychoanalysis (various types);
- insight-directed psychotherapy; and
- supportive psychotherapy.

and depending on the therapist, you can expect a mixture of Freud, behaviourism, Adler, Maslow, Jung, Horney, Fromm,

Erikson—even Maharishi or Zen philosophy thrown in. If you're well enough when you're referred (and if you care!), you can try grilling the therapist on what theories he or she draws upon and how they are supposed to work.

Among all the confusion and clamour, there are a few basic principles common to many psychotherapies:

- the Self naturally moves towards its own growth;
- emotional insight is important to this growth;
- growth is achieved through the relationship between the therapist and the client.[9]

You'll also want to know how the sessions work and what the rules are about cancelling appointments (some therapists charge the full consultation rate if you don't come, and Medicare won't rebate a single cent). Just as importantly, find out what to expect emotionally during the course of therapy. Will you be settled enough to go to work after a morning session? Also find out roughly how long the therapy should take—some therapists aim to do a quick, intense intervention over weeks or months while others are in it for the long haul.

Of course, the type and duration of therapy depends rather a lot on what it is that you are having problems with. (Or what the referring doctor thinks is wrong with you.) Get as clear a picture as you can from the referring doctor as to what they think needs to be fixed. If you think this particular thing 'ain't broke' you are within your rights to insist that it not be 'fixed'. (You are the customer and yours is the hand that signs the cheque.)

Once you meet the therapist, try to judge if it is a good thing to go ahead. If you're an intuitive type, use your intuition but also use your eyes and ears. If you usually rely on objective data, add the information you get from your gut.

Mostly, once you've committed to this kind of therapy, you're stuck with it for the duration the therapist indicated. If you want out, you'll find the therapist could be extremely persuasive and insistent that you stay in. In some instances, this could actually be good doctoring—if you drop out of therapy at a particular stage, you could be extremely emotionally vulnerable and even quite confused because the changes you wanted to make through therapy may be incomplete.

Not everyone has the sort of problems that can be helped with psychotherapy. Typically this sort of therapy is said to be the best for people with long-term issues such as personality disturbances, or survivors of major life trauma in addition to manic depression. On top of that, you have to be able to afford the time and the money involved, and you have to be reasonably articulate, as the effectiveness of therapy relies on your ability in using language. Before you sign up, make sure you understand what the referring doctor thinks about:

- your current diagnosis;
- how well the treatment so far has helped;
- how much better he or she thinks you can get with the proposed therapy;
- what sort of psychotherapy he or she thinks you need;
- exactly how that psychotherapy is expected to work;
- how long the therapy is expected to last—weeks, months or years;
- how much time and money commitment is expected of you;
- whether there is another suspected diagnosis in addition to the diagnosis you've been told about;
- what is expected to happen to your condition(s) if you do not take up psychotherapy; and
- what alternatives are there.

Supportive/problem-solving counselling

'Counselling' covers a wide range of activities from being central to our treatment to occasional sessions for solving specific problems.

If you're functioning well on a day-to-day level, the less indepth approaches of counselling techniques might be all you need. Like psychotherapists, counsellors offer a wide variety of types of help. Most prefer to use 'non-directive' styles, where the client makes his or her own discoveries. Where there are pressing matters, a more 'directive' style might be used, or the session could be used for joint problem-solving. You'll usually be able to negotiate the number of sessions you'll have, and set the goals for the counselling at the start. Choose a counsellor on recommendation, qualification and, above all, their trust and respect of you.

Peer support and counselling

Increasingly, community and other services for people with mental illness are providing peer support programs. These vary widely in their approach and level of formality, but are generally based on the assumption that if a counsellor shares our perspective and experience, their approach will be more empathetic. Peer support activities can be tracked down via mental health services and consumer organisations (see Appendix II).

Family therapy

Family therapy, conducted by your treating psychiatrist or another mental health worker, can be a useful way of educating immediate family members in an atmosphere that is reasonably controlled (it's less likely to degenerate into a blaming-bloodbath with an outsider present). Wait until you're well before you attempt it. If you're worried that you might be 'ganged up on', seek assurances from the worker that he or she will make sure everyone is safe. Plan an escape mechanism, or arrange to bring a trusted friend with you.

If you have a 'double trouble' issue that involves your family (for example, childhood sexual abuse or family violence), tread carefully and be guided by people outside the family (that is, psychiatrist, friends).

Your confidentiality must be maintained by all those involved. Psychiatrists hardly ever break a patient's confidentiality, to do so could lead to him or her losing their registration to practice. But family members have no such deterrent.

When I overdosed, I was taken to the hospital where my mother works as a nurse on the surgical ward... Later I discovered that she had managed to get access to my medical record. When you're ill you lose all your privileges as an adult.

Debbie

Positive outcomes of family therapy can include:

- family members' recognition of early warning signs;
- agreement on when family members should take action;
- fresh agreement about everyone's role and expectations of each other;
- agreement on how and in what circumstances family members should contact the psychiatrist; and
- making of joint 'Safety Nets' and 'Brakes' (see Chapter 9);
- family members' education about confidentiality and securing their agreement to maintain your right to have medical information remain confidential.[10]

The deep-and-meaningful

Deep-and-meaningful, and its close cousin whingeing, is the treatment most of us seek first. There is no stigma attached, nor is there a fee. There's no risk of being prescribed medicine or locked up and you can be reasonably sure that the person you talk to will be sympathetic and won't rock the boat of your belief that you're basically okay.

Choose carefully the person with whom you indulge in whinge or deep-and-meaningful sessions. Can you afford to lose them if they start to feel swamped? Are they motivated by care for you or the chance to give advice? Do you *want* an opportunity to tell them to get packing by surreptitiously seeking, then rejecting, their advice? All people, no matter how close you are initially, will be burned by too much neediness. Okay, from time to time we are needy (that's a statement of fact, not a criticism), but friends have their own responsibilities and may well feel inadequate or impotent to help you. The end result can be loss of otherwise good friends.

Some people simply have no idea what it is to suffer—their life experience hasn't delivered that knowledge to them. Don't expect them to understand—in fact, expect them to tell you, like one friend told me, 'You don't need all these drugs. You should be able to do it yourself. Just pull yourself together.' My options boiled down to either walk away or snot her in the face or shrug and try to stay friends, allowing for her myopic attitude. Since then I've been careful to open up only to people whose own life experience has taught them compassion.

Who should know and how much should you tell them?

Be careful who you tell that you're seeing a counsellor or therapist, and what you talk about. Lots of people appear to be helpful and empathic but underneath they're terrified, want to feel good by giving advice, or even want us to give them enough information so they can use it against us.

If people around are intrusive, wanting to know a word-by-word description of every session, it's often hard to deny them. But even if they aren't just being voyeuristic, this intrusiveness can lead to a feeling of the counselling or therapy being undermined. If it's causing you problems, speak to the counsellor or therapist about it—it's a common 'unwanted effect'.

At the other end of the scale is people's apparent indifference. Keeping your talking therapy separate can be useful, but there may be times that a change you're considering making will impact on your relationship and you might want to explain how you arrived at your decision to make that change. Apparent indifference can mask all sorts of things, such as mistrust of the counselling or therapy, or feeling that the person is losing intimacy with you because you have 'secrets' with someone else. Again, if it's causing a problem, discuss it with the counsellor or therapist.

COMPLEMENTARY AND ALTERNATIVE THERAPIES

For most of us, maximising our well-being involves taking medicine and participating in talking therapies. However, Western psychiatry is increasingly being seen as offering only an incomplete range of approaches, with its reliance on medicine and biological explanations for the phenomena of mental illness.

People with manic depression are increasingly taking the best of conventional psychiatry's offerings and seeking out complementary or alternative healers. However, I've found that many alternative practitioners seem to be scared of me or my symptoms and/or are not trained or prepared to use their modality for healing of mental illness.

Some alternative healing modalities are discussed below.

Meditation, yoga, contemplative exercise

Meditation, yoga and the gentle movements of Eastern 'exercises' take many forms. Some people have told me that meditation can exacerbate depression but others benefit from the practice.

Early Western meditation techniques included the Jacobsen method, a routine used in many antenatal classes. This involves progressively contracting the muscles of the extremities and relaxing them until your body warms, fuzzes and lifts a little.

Many Eastern techniques use a mantra—a special sound or word that resonates with your mind, body and soul. A method well known in the West is Transcendental Meditation, or TM®.[11] The routine here is twenty minutes in the morning and the early evening. A mantra is selected for you by your teacher.

You focus without effort on the mantra as you sit quietly, eyes closed. From time to time thoughts come in—these are said to represent the stress that is leaving your body. Effortlessly you return to the mantra. Eventually you 'lose' the mantra—a sign of 'transcending', and a peacefulness and bliss comes to you that is simply breathtaking. Afterwards, you feel grounded, relaxed and quietly powerful.[12]

Yoga and Tai Chi are other powerful ways to improve well-being. Try to achieve a level of commitment that's not too high—and not too low—to enable you to stick at the technique you choose for a reasonable period.

Reiki

Reiki, Japanese for 'universal life energy', draws on that energy to enhance the healing effects of other healing modalities.[13] Deeply relaxing, reiki can settle much of the distress of a manic-depressive episode, often very quickly taking the heat out of a crisis. The reiki practioner may use other healing techniques in conjunction with reiki, such as massage and aromatherapy. Reiki is a so-called 'energetic' healing process that reconnects us to the energy of the universe. The healer's hands are placed gently on or just away from the body at key points known as 'chakras', the body's energy centres. Reiki healers and teachers can be found in private practice around Australia.

Aromatherapy

This involves using essential oils either on the skin, burning them in water, in a bath and so on. Some essential oils appear to have both calming and antidepressant effects. See Table 5.4.

You can try out some of the oils on their own or mix and match them according to your needs, although there are some combinations that should be avoided. For detailed information consult one of the many books on the subject or seek advice from a specialist aromatherapist.

Homeopathy

Homeopathy looks to the underlying cause of illness and assesses the patient holistically. Doses of medicines are taken in small quantities. Although homeopathy is hampered by the use of other drugs, a homeopath may be able to give you a remedy with which you can reduce your dose of prescribed medicines. Be careful and let both your psychiatrist and the homeopath know what is happening.[14]

Herbal remedies

Herbal medicine is another holistic discipline. It uses herbs and plants to assist natural healing. St John's Wort (*Hypericum perforatum*) is increasingly being used for its antidepressant action. The active ingredient, hypericin, works in a similar way as monoamine oxidase inhibitors (MAOIs—see Chapter 4) and, like them, can take a few weeks to have effect. There is a potential for drug interactions between some prescribed medicines and St John's Wort, so discuss the matter with the doctor who prescribed the other medicine.

Herbal remedies are also useful for improving our general health in between major episodes.[15]

Problem	Category of oil	Examples of oils
Depression	Antidepressant oils	Angelica, basil, bergamot, Roman chamomile, clary sage, frankincense, geranium, grapefruit, jasmine, lavender, lemon, mandarin, neroli, orange, rose, sandalwood, ylang ylang.
Hypomania Agitation Anxiety Panic Sleep	Sedative oils	Basil, Roman chamomile, clary, sage, everlasting, jasmine, lavender, mandarin, French marjoram, neroli, sandalwood, ylang ylang.

Table 5.4 Aromatherapy in manic depression

Chinese medicine including acupuncture

Acupuncture and other forms of traditional Chinese medicine can be effective to help maintain health between episodes.[16]

Chiropractic

There is some anecdotal evidence that cerebral adjustment, a specialist technique, can be useful in healing the symptoms of manic depression.

Body work

Somatic psychotherapy, body work or somatotherapy are some of the terms used to describe techniques for integrating awareness and healing of your body with healing of 'mind' issues. The techniques can be especially useful if you have a background of trauma or abuse. Practitioners may have no recognised qualifications (be careful) or be very highly qualified (for example, a Masters degree in psychology plus qualifications in somatic therapy and/or massage etc.).

Cathartic therapies and therapies based on the arts

I include here art therapy, music therapy, dance therapy, psychodrama and also those 'personal growth' weekend workshops on account of their cathartic impact. Attractive because they are short and sharp, these therapies have in common the technique of expression of the subconscious through the art form being used.

Although it can be said that most legitimate therapies can be beneficial, hypnosis, psychodrama and some of the more cathartic approaches can sometimes place us in danger. I came a bit unravelled during a group class in which the teacher drew on techniques of spiritual practice and art therapy. I found myself painting straight from my subconscious, creating images of scenes I would not recognise for a number of years to come. Because I couldn't integrate what I was painting, I became distressed and somewhat preoccupied with the images. I do not wish to malign any of these therapeutic approaches but merely to reiterate their potential hazards to people with certain vulnerabilities. So if you're considering doing hypnosis, psychodrama, primal therapy or certain sorts of intense group work, check it out with your mainstream/Western psychiatric service provider first, and weigh up the various opinions.

SUPPORT AND EDUCATION GROUPS

Finding people who understand some of our experiences and whose perspective on life is similar to our own can be like a 'coming home'. They may be found in chance meetings of individuals or organised formally in community groups for self-help, support, education or advocacy. Among such people we can often find a comfortable, familiar and safe space from which to draw strength for recovery. Details of some of these groups appear in Appendix II.

6

GETTING THE BEST AND AVOIDING THE WORST

FINDING A GOOD PSYCHIATRIST

I attended a psychiatrist, Dr R, for a couple of years in my late teens. He had a waiting room with about fifteen or twenty chairs and it was always full. When I first went there I had to wait over an hour and assumed there had been some emergency that had called the doctor away. But it turned out to be the norm; in fact, a wait of two or three hours was usual. Only years later when I had developed a sense of self worth did I realise how arrogant and abusive this practice had been. If that happened to me now I would most certainly complain.

Therese

There *is* such a thing as a good psychiatrist—and most of us find one sooner or later. But there are many different ideas as to what exactly makes a psychiatrist a 'good psychiatrist'. You might want above all else someone you can really communicate with; someone who listens; someone who doesn't tell you what to do but is prepared to give advice; someone who is prepared to 'carry the can' in a crisis; or someone who has time for a chat or a joke. You might find it important to be able to negotiate fees if you're off work. Or to have someone who is available after hours. Or someone who doesn't keep you waiting too long. Alternatively, you might place primary importance on someone who specialises in manic depression or who has a reputation of being expert at medication.

I think there is only one good way to find a psychiatrist who fits our criteria: by chance. This, after all, is how most of us find our spouse!

We can improve our chances in a number of ways.

- Get referred by a general practitioner who you trust and who knows you well.
- Identify exactly what aspects are most important (for example, trust and communication; reputation; specialisation in manic depression etc.) and let the general practitioner or other psychiatrist know.
- Put a toe in the water by seeking a second opinion. This way, if you like the new psychiatrist you have the option of switching: if you don't, you still have your original psychiatrist in the mean time.

Some words of caution:

- A psychiatrist who holds a senior academic or hospital appointment doesn't necessarily have above average competence in actually healing people.
- A private psychiatrist will not necessarily refuse to bulk-bill you.
- You can ask another of the psychiatrist's patients what they think, but you have to meet the other patient first because the psychiatrist won't give out the names of patients. Be wary, as the other patient might have different ideas from yours about what makes a 'good psychiatrist'.
- Don't be too hasty to judge the psychiatrist.

It's always difficult to know when or if we should switch doctors. Like any long-term, intimate relationship, it can seem too much like hard work to start all over again with someone new. It's hard to tell whether we should just work harder at the existing relationship or risk throwing out the baby with the bath water.

The questions in Table 6.1 are designed to prompt your thinking about your psychiatrist as you might with any important relationship.

IMPROVING THE EFFECTIVENESS OF TREATMENT

Psychiatrists are human just like us. I imagine they have a 'wish list' that spells out the sort of patient they like most to work with.

> *Psychiatrists are motivated by the patient who is motivated to get well.*

Obviously, if your psychiatrist is motivated, your experience of treatment and even its outcome will be improved. To improve the performance of your psychiatrist and the effectiveness of treatment, simply try to motivate the psychiatrist. Psychiatrist Bertie Schrinken (not his real name) is motivated by patients who:

- want to be well;
- ask him questions;
- are motivated to take medicine if needed;
- want to make joint decisions about treatment;
- don't get cross when he has to point out that they are being self-defeating; and
- do their best to work on their non-medical problems.

HOW TO READ A PRESCRIPTION

There was a saying at university that students were chosen for the medical course on the basis of their unintelligible writing—then they were taught for six years to make it

What seems to be the problem?	What can you do about it?	Relevant facts
Is it impossible to get to appointments because of timing or location?	Talk to the psychiatrist and explain.	Sometimes the psychiatrist can give you appointments at a better time of day. If not, they're usually happy to refer in this situation.
Has communication broken down?	First, attend to your side of the breakdown—these things are rarely one-sided. Talk with the psychiatrist about your joint problem. If you still feel you're not being listened to, get a referral to a different psychiatrist. Tell the first psychiatrist what you're doing and why.	Psychiatrists have a gentleman's agreement not to 'poach' one another's patients. Even if you want to see Shrink 2, Shrink 2 won't see you unless you have severed ties with Shrink 1. Shrink 2 will write to Shrink 1 and dob you in. This practice has one benefit: it helps minimise our chances of being prescribed conflicting medicine or other treatment by more than one doctor.

Table 6.1 Some common problems in people's relationship with their psychiatrist

What seems to be the problem?		Relevant facts
Do you feel you're getting nowhere?	Tread carefully. Sometimes a major breakthrough comes just after a period of feeling as if you're stagnating. It can take years to bring manic depression under control, and a long-term relationship with a psychiatrist means you can build a strong team that can supply safety nets and brakes when needed.	Don't go 'doctor shopping'—it results in 'care chopping' and an ever-worsening sense that you're not making progress.
Has the psychiatrist behaved inappropriately?	Seek (from another doctor) immediate referral to another psychiatrist. Get counselling if needed from outside the medical profession or mental health service. Is a complaint warranted? Some avenues for complaint are listed in Appendix III.	Inappropriate sexual or other behaviour from someone as crucial as your psychiatrist can set you back years if you let it. Get onto some impartial advice. Don't excuse the psychiatrist's behaviour on the grounds that you're feeling too unwell or insecure to change doctors.

Table 6.1 cont Some common problems in people's relationship with their psychiatrist

illegible as well. Jokes aside, the legibility of prescriptions is important. For example, the Medical Practitioners' Board of Victoria conducted an informal hearing in 1996 into a complaint against a doctor who had written an illegible prescription. The doctor was forced to acknowledge 'that in the event that pharmacists are ... unable to decipher hand written prescriptions, the public may be placed at risk.'[1]

Many doctors now use computers to print prescriptions. The software they use also allows them to make sure the drug won't cause you harm by cross-checking the prescribed drug against other conditions you might have or medicines you're taking.

Problems of actual illegibility aside, it's useful to be able to interpret scripts. Consider this fictional-but-all-too-possible case.

Sharon, who takes carbamazepine for manic depression, needed to go back on the oral contraceptive pill. Sharon gets a script for the Pill and reads it as she leaves the consulting room. She notices it's the standard-strength (30 mg) pill she used to take before she started carbamazepine. Sharon had heard that carbamazepine reduces the reliability of the Pill, so she heads back to the doctor and the mistake is rectified.

Whew! What if she hadn't noticed? A surprise pregnancy could have been on the cards, with risks from the carbamazepine to Sharon and her baby. It's true that the doctor is responsible for what he or she prescribes, but I prefer to exercise my own responsibility as well when it comes to critical issues like my health! Figure 6.1 illustrates some of the conventional Latin and abbreviations used in prescriptions.

HOSPITAL

In the fairly recent past, hospital stays of several weeks or even months were typical in the experience of people with manic depression. This afforded intensive, 24-hour treatment and

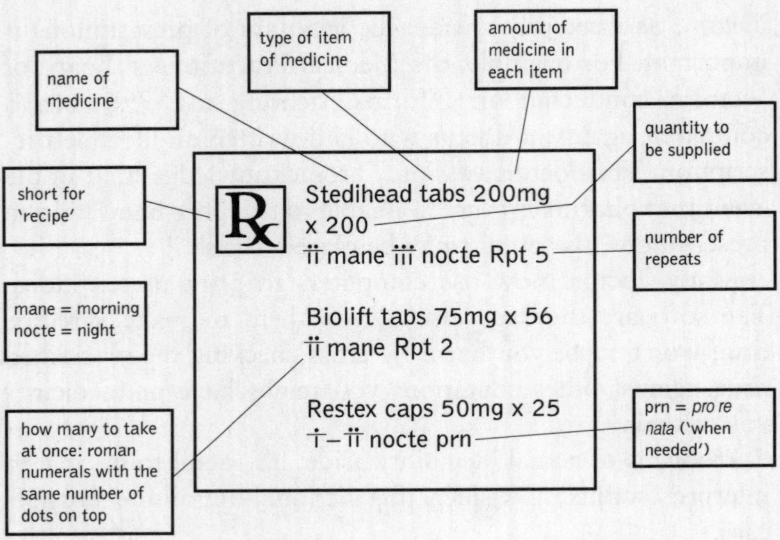

Figure 6.1 How to interpret a prescription

safety from the extremes of illness, time to learn about managing our lives, and refuge from those social situations that make it harder to recover.

Progressive mental health legislation in most Australian States enshrines the principle of giving necessary care and treatment in the 'least restrictive environment'.[2] This ideology, operating hand-in-hand with the imperative to reduce costs of hospitalisation, led to a revolution in hospital care during the 1990s. Hospitalisation is now a minimalist service, focussing on containment of dangerous behaviour and the quick suppression of the worst symptoms. The average length of stay in public hospitals has been steadily dropping. In Victoria, for example, hospitals are aiming to reduce the average stay by half—to just eight days. Public hospitals now confess privately to discharging people who are still 'acutely ill' back to community treatment. People who are still suffering severe symptoms are often discharged to sub-standard crisis accommodation. Community-based treatment varies greatly, but immediately after discharge it may consist at best of daily visiting services and crisis assessment services.

Private hospitals have tended to offer longer inpatient stays, but are coming under increasing pressure from health insurance companies to reduce the length of stay. Unlike people who use the public system, those who use private hospitals are not usually able to access publicly run community visiting services after being discharged.

What to expect in hospital

Nothing can prepare a person for the psychological impact of being admitted to a psychiatric hospital, but there are some strategies for making the stay a little easier. Experienced people know that in hospital it is wise to expect the worst and be prepared. The best source of information is other patients. House rules and routines are rarely written down and we discover what they are by inadvertently breaking them and enduring the consequences. More importantly, we learn very quickly that expressions of extreme anger, frustration, despair or joy are actively discouraged and often punished. The following is an amalgam of various rules of thumb that experienced patients have discovered.

Routines and rules

NECESSITIES Getting access to tobacco and toiletries is sometimes a problem in hospital. Find out from other patients where the nearest shop is and how and when patients can go there.

MEALS Most kitchens are closed between meal times and there may or may not be snacks such as fruit available when the kitchen is closed. Find out what the meal times are if you don't want to miss out. Morning and afternoon tea and supper are often served, but watch out for the extra calories. The combination of being in hospital doing less physical activity, psychiatric medicine and extra food make hospital a dangerous place if you're concerned about your weight.

Tea and coffee-making facilities are usually freely available in hospital, but if you're having difficulty sleeping or resting, watch your caffeine intake (it's a stimulant) and ask for decaffeinated coffee or herbal tea.

ACTIVITIES Activities available in public psychiatric hospitals are typically limited to smoking and watching television. If you're lucky, there may be facilities such as pool, table tennis, board games, stereo, CDs and maybe a piano or art materials. There may even be an occupational therapist attached to the ward who organises activities, but this is becoming less likely in public hospitals. If you can concentrate, bring a book or learn to like daytime television. Hospitals tend to offer the 'lowest stimulus environment' so as not to add to our difficulties. However, if you've been hospitalised during a period of mania, you'll know that boredom tends to exacerbate the distress. Keep as active as you can—walk, run, do pushups, improvise a cricket or handball game—and try to keep out of trouble. Private hospitals have a wider range of activities, mainly organised by occupational therapists.

STAFF ROUTINES The working day of hospital staff is based on three shifts. It's worth finding out the times of the shifts, so if you need to, you can catch up with a particular staff member before they knock off. At the end of each shift, the nursing staff 'hand over' to the new shift in a closed session in the staff office. In handover, nurses are expected to describe to the new shift any current issues affecting their patients. Interruptions to handover are viewed dimly by staff and experienced hospital patients learn to avoid requesting any assistance during these sessions.

LAUNDRY Most hospitals have free laundry facilities. Ask other patients where the laundry is and about the routine. An iron might be available but for safety reasons will be kept under staff supervision.

DRESS CODE Staff and patients alike these days wear comfortable street clothes during the day. Some hospitals still insist that you wear standard-issue flannelette pyjamas ('prison greens') if you don't have a change of clothes, and you can make a formal complaint about this, but be careful of being victimised afterwards.

Psychiatric hospitals can be dangerous places and I'd strongly suggest that you don't wear clothing that is revealing or sexually provocative.

TELEPHONE Many hospitals have public telephones which can receive incoming calls. Ask other patients what the incoming number is so you can give it to family and friends. Patients share the job of answering the phone and locating the person being called.

Outgoing calls can usually be made, but staff may or may not be prepared to exchange coins for you to use the phone.

VISITORS Formal visiting hours are becoming a thing of the past. However, it's best to ask your visitors to phone first to make sure you'll be available. You have the right to refuse any or all visitors. If you want to refuse visitors, tell a staff member and ask him or her to convey that to the visitor.

Children aren't prohibited, but because of the potentially scary environment (there are usually no separate visiting areas) many parents decide not to have their children visit.

LEAVING THE WARD If you are an 'voluntary' patient, you are notionally free to use all of the grounds in the hospital. However, as the hospital is responsible for the well-being of all its patients, staff expect you to let them know of your intentions.

If you are in a public hospital as an involuntary ('committed') patient, you must get staff approval to leave the immediate ward area. If you do leave the area without approval, staff will assume you are absconding and you are likely to be chased, tackled, locked up in seclusion and given a sedative injection in your behind.

POSSESSIONS AND MONEY If you have any valuables including cash, let your contact nurse know as soon as possible after arriving. Hospitals may hold patients' money in trust. You should be given a receipt for your possessions/cash and may be asked to sign a waiver. The waiver means that you give up your right to sue the hospital if your possessions/cash are damaged or lost. Because of this, it is in your best interest to have any valuables taken home, or to another safe place.

Sometimes 'glitches' occur in the social security system if you are receiving payments when you come into hospital. Let the hospital's social worker know as soon as possible if this happens to you.

The hospital has a responsibility to make sure there are no dangerous items on the ward and staff may check your possessions and temporarily confiscate medicines, belts, knives, razor blades and electrical equipment.

BED TIME, GETTING UP TIME Most hospitals have routine times for getting up and going to bed. Some even lock patients out of their bedrooms during the day. The best source of information about this is other patients.

LOCKING POLICY Most wards are locked overnight in the same way you'd lock a house up for the night. Very few general acute psychiatric wards are still locked during the day.

Avoiding danger

RESTRAINT 'Restraint' refers to means of subduing people whose mental state renders them a danger to themselves or others. The usual process is physical restraint ('nursing staff holding patients for their [sic] own protection'[3]) followed by chemical restraint (administration of discretionary doses of prescribed medicine, usually by intramuscular injection).

Mechanical restraint can also be used, involving strapping a patient to a bed to prevent movement.[4]

SECLUSION 'Seclusion' is the

> temporary isolation and detention of a person in a locked room if they are behaving in a way which is disruptive, violent or potentially dangerous to themselves, other patients, or staff. To minimise risk to the person, the typical seclusion room has no fittings and resembles a prison cell, with a small reinforced viewing window.[5]

Seclusion rooms can appear inhumane, and the practice of seclusion is at best a nursing practice of last resort; at worst a means of punishment and banishment.

Experienced patients are divided on their opinions of seclusion. Angela said, 'Seclusion's got its place, as long as it's used properly. It gets you away from the chaos of the ward.'

Another person said:

> They put me in seclusion for three days once, with a mattress, a blanket and a bedpan. They brought me food, but they hardly ever checked on me. It was awful. There wasn't any light.

The experience of seclusion can create a variety of responses in patients and staff alike:

> They put me in there and I started banging on the door. They ignored me, of course. So I started unravelling the carpet, picked at it 'til it started unravelling. I unravelled about a quarter of it before they came and got me. That's why they pulled up the carpet and there's only the concrete floor there now.
>
> Frank

The only advice for survival in such a situation is to appear to be calm and happy to comply with whatever is asked of you—or avoid getting put in seclusion in the first place.

'HIGH DEPENDENCY' 'High dependency' is both a physical space and a style of nursing. It is not regulated by legislation. High dependency typically comprises a sparse, locked common area onto which open lockable seclusion rooms and possibly larger, unlocked bedrooms. Staff work inside a reinforced glass cubicle or office.

People are placed in a high dependency area for a wide variety of reasons, ranging from simply being upset to being violent, out of control, suicidal, at risk of self-harm or even because they need protection from other patients.

Experienced patients learn to refrain from 'making waves' in high dependency.

SPECIALLING The nursing practice of 'specialling' involves assigning a nurse to keep within very close contact with a patient for the entire shift. When done well, patients assessed are able to benefit from the close attention and it can be a very effective means of healing. However, the experience of many people who've been 'specialled' is that it is like having a personal prison warden scrutinise their every move. Good specialling, where the nurse is prepared to listen constructively and empathically and to convey his or her respect for the patient, is rare. Further, because specialling is an expensive use of nursing resources, the practice appears to be diminishing.

OTHER PATIENTS Living with a group of strangers is difficult at the best of times and in hospital personal space is at a premium. Some of our most rewarding friendships are made in hospital and the contact with other patients can be healing. However, not every contact is rewarding, and you need to be wary of interactions with people on the ward that could be damaging—particularly where you want to help other patients. If you find yourself being distressed by another patient's story, tactfully get yourself out of the situation—it's the nurses' job, not yours, to help people resolve their difficulties.

SEXUAL ASSAULT Assault and sexual assault are critical issues for many patients, as Simon told me:

> I had just got into hospital after being flown home from WA. I was a mess. All I wanted to do was lie on my bed. A couple of days later this woman patient came into my room and raped me. The staff did nothing.

The Burdekin inquiry[6] found that this was not an isolated case. Assault and sexual assault on staff by patients, among patients, and on patients by staff all took place.

As a hospital patient you have the same rights as people outside hospital to disclose or not disclose sexual assault and you have the right, but cannot be forced, to report it to the police.

PROTECT YOUR SECRETS Many, if not most, people with a mental illness have events in their recent or distant past which are directly relevant to their current experience of distress. However, because the focus of hospital treatment is quick reduction of the most distressing symptoms, staff often pay little attention to healing the effects of past events.

In hospital, you can use the availability of nurses to talk about and try to heal previous trauma. However, this can and does cause unwanted consequences, such as a dismissive response or even a longer stay or increased medication. On the other hand, good nursing, even over a short period, can give us new resources for our quest for healing.

COPING WITH DISRESPECT The single most important element in a hospital for the well-being of patients is respect from staff,[7] but my advice is to expect the opposite and be prepared to be tolerant. Basic human courtesy from staff can be rare in hospital. Disrespect is entrenched in more complex interactions, such as having to attend 'ward rounds' in which ten or more staff discuss your case in front of you, or having to cope alone with the impact of having been physically restrained or secluded.

Everyone can get angry if they are treated disrespectfully and people in hospital are no exception. However, people in psychiatric hospitals are typically victimised if they express outrage at outrageous treatment. Most people I have spoken to agree that to survive in hospital you're better off if you can 'play the game', swallow your pride and bite your tongue. You can always make a complaint after you've been discharged.

PRIVATE VS PUBLIC Top quality psychiatric care can be had in either the public or private mental health sectors—and each sector has its human rights shortfalls. All that differs is the emphasis on a number of points, which are outlined in Table 6.2.

Typical features	Private	Public
Accommodation	Ranges from ★★★ to ★★★★★ Private and shared rooms, generally with ensuite bathrooms. Common areas may or may not be gender-segregated.	Ranges from ★★ to ★★★★ Private and shared rooms with bathrooms. Newer facilities may have ensuites. Common areas may or may not be gender-segregated.
Compulsory admission	No	Compulsory or voluntary
Voluntary admission	Yes	Yes, although rare
Users of service are called	Patients	Clients, Consumers
Cost	Depends on your level of health insurance. Very few people can afford to do without insurance and pay cash. Up-front payment may be requested.	Free
Outdoor access, facilities	Usually some outdoor access to gardens or 'courtyards'; low security.	Older hospitals may have large grounds; newer facilities have small 'courtyards'. Outdoor access may be limited.
Type of condition treated	Anxiety conditions, depression, obsessive-compulsive disorder, post-traumatic stress, life crises, alcohol and drug rehabilitation, post-natal psychosis/depression, manic depression, schizophrenia.	'Serious mental illness'—schizophrenia, manic depression. Recent attempts to expand 'seriousness of condition' to include other disorders, for example anxiety, personality disorders.

Table 6.2 A comparison of private and public hospitals

Typical features	Private	Public
Type of programs	Mother-and-baby, cognitive-behavioural and/or supportive talking therapy, occupational therapy, relaxation, social work, psychology. No case management.	Treatment mainly focused on medicine. Social workers and case managers may be involved. May or may not have occupational therapy, relaxation, psychology.
Locked wards	Not legally	Yes, although not in all hospitals.
Length of stay	Longer than public hospitals. Length of stay influenced by health insurers' policies.	Short and decreasing. Length of stay influenced by State's health department policies.
ECT	Yes, if licensed.	Yes, if licensed.
Seclusion	None known	Yes
Post discharge arrangements	Via admitting psychiatrist and/or social worker and/or family members	Via admitting psychiatrist and/or case worker and/or social worker and/or accommodation worker and/or general practitioner and/or family members
Policy and development	Continual, guided by National Mental Health Strategy; not answerable to State health departments except for specified issues, such as ECT licensing.	Continual, largely driven by State health departments and National Mental Health Strategy. Includes projects such as Consumer Participation, Shared Care with GPs, outcome measurement, etc.

7

RIGHTS, TREATMENT AND THE LAW

Much madness is divinest sense
To a discerning eye;
Much sense the starkest madness.
'T is the majority
In this, as all, prevails.
Assent, and you are sane;
Demur, you're straightaway dangerous,
And handled with a chain.

Emily Dickinson

Staying out of trouble with the law for us involves this maxim: First, know the rules, then play by them.

Many a hospital patient has gone for an innocent stroll in leafy hospital grounds, only to be sprinted after and rugby-tackled by three massive male nurses. The nurses fear that we might abscond; we expect to be able to use the grounds of the hospital as part of our healing journey.

Others have been caught in a more insidious trap: knowing they have to collect medicine at certain times, they get held up with a consultation with a psychiatrist. This is then interpreted as a refusal of medication and the hapless voluntary patient becomes involuntary, with all the loss of freedoms that status means.

It's not just in hospital where we can get into trouble because of the want of knowing the rules. Any dealing with the police—as a victim of crime, a perpetrator, even on traffic matters—can suddenly become frighteningly hazardous. Many people, without knowing that the police have the right, are justifiably upset when the police break into their homes and cart them off under suspicion of being mentally ill and a danger to themselves or others.

Getting in and out of trouble with the law is too often part and parcel of having manic depression, but we can limit the damage by knowing our rights and responsibilities, and the responsibilities of police and psychiatric hospitals. We can also use the law to remedy situations where we've sustained some damage. In this chapter we'll look at the law relating to treatment by mental health services and dealing with police. Aspects of law relating to employment, money and education are dealt with in the relevant chapters. This chapter is intended only as a general outline of the law and if you want to rely on advice on any aspect of the law you should see a solicitor, community legal centre or mental health legal service.

- Know your rights and responsibilities.
- Assert your rights now if you can.
- Bide your time and make sure you survive to fight later if you have to.

LEGAL AND POLICY FRAMEWORK

International principles

The United Nations Declaration on Human Rights of 1948 is the fundamental document on human rights throughout the world. There are some 30 statements in it dealing with legal and political rights, the rights of children, race rights and so on. The Declaration is the document upon which most equal opportunity legislation in Australia is based.

In 1978, the World Health Organisation's International Conference on Primary Health Care issued a declaration (Declaration of Alma-Ata[1]) that spells out certain principles for health, including 'health, which is a state of complete physical, mental and social well-being… is a fundamental human right' and that 'people have the right and duty to participate individually and collectively in the planning and implementation of their health care'.

The two Declarations are applied in the United Nations Principles for the Protection of Persons with Mental Illness and for the Improvement of Mental Health Care.

Australian Government policy

A Statement of Mental Health Rights and Responsibilities was adopted by Australian Health Ministers in 1991 which has formed part of the development of subsequent policies such as the National Mental Health Policy (1992), the National Mental Health Plans (1992, 1998) and National Standards for Mental Health Services (1996).

Consumer and advocacy organisations

The International Year of the Disabled (1981) saw the birth of state funding for groups of people with disabilities. Since then, the Australian Mental Health Consumers' Network has been established. Western Australia and Victoria have legal centres with a specific focus on mental health law.

There are also a number of disability discrimination and advocacy services in all States and Territories. For contact details see Appendix III.

MENTAL HEALTH SERVICES

All States have legislation governing how mental health services are delivered and some give explicit rights to people with a mental illness. Some of the key features are compared overleaf.

Purpose and principles

In New South Wales, the Australian Capital Territory, South Australia, Western Australia, Tasmania and Victoria, mental health legislation is based on access to the best standard of care and treatment with minimum restriction on people's rights and liberty. Queensland and Northern Territory legislation is based on the older principles of custody and guardianship, although the Queensland Parliament is considering a bill to reform that State's mental health legislation.

Compulsory treatment

Criteria for being compulsorily treated in hospital are spelled out in all legislation. The most 'user-friendly' are the criteria in use in Victoria and Western Australia, as they specify that compulsory treatment only applies where you haven't given your consent and where there are no less restrictive alternatives to hospitalisation. As a general guide, these are the criteria you have to address if you want to get out of compulsory treatment.

New South Wales 'If the person is suffering from mental illness and, owing to that illness, there are reasonable grounds for believing that care, treatment or control of the person is necessary:

(a) for the person's own protection from serious harm, or
(b) for the protection of others from serious harm.'[2]

Australian Capital Territory 'Where a doctor... believes on reasonable grounds that:

(a) a person is mentally dysfunctional and, as a consequence, requires immediate treatment or care;
(b) the person has refused to receive that treatment or care;
(c) detention is necessary for the person's own health or safety or for the protection of members of the public; and
(d) adequate treatment or care cannot be provided in a less restrictive environment.'[3]

Victoria 'If

(a) the person appears to be mentally ill; and
(b) the person's mental illness requires immediate treatment and that treatment can be obtained by admission ... ; and
(c) because of the person's mental illness, the person should be admitted ... for treatment ... for his or her health or safety ... or for the protection of members of the public; and
(d) the person has refused or is unable to consent to the necessary treatment for the mental illness; and
(e) the person cannot receive adequate treatment ... in a manner less restrictive of that person's freedom of decision and action.'[4]

Tasmania 'If

(a) the person appears to have a mental illness; and
(b) there is, in consequence, a significant risk of harm to the person or others; and
(c) the detention of the person as an involuntary patient is necessary to protect the person or others; and
(d) the approved hospital is properly equipped and staffed for the care or treatment of the person.'[5]

South Australia 'If, after examining a person, a medical practitioner is satisfied:

(a) that the person has a mental illness that requires immediate treatment; and
(b) that such treatment is available in an approved treatment centre; and
(c) that the person should be admitted ... in the interests of his or her own health and safety or for the protection of other persons.'[6]

Western Australia 'Only if:

(a) the person has a mental illness requiring treatment;
(b) the treatment can be provided through detention in an authorized hospital or through a community treatment order and is required to be so provided in order:

(i) to protect the health or safety of that person or any other person;
(ii) to protect the person from self-inflicted harm ... ;
(iii) to prevent the person doing serious damage to any property;

(c) the person has refused, or due to the nature of the mental illness, is unable to consent to treatment; and
(d) the treatment cannot be adequately provided in a way that would involve less restriction of the freedom of choice and movement of the person ... '[7]

Northern Territory 'Where a medical practitioner ... or a member of the Police Force has reasonable cause to believe that a person:

(a) by reason of a mental illness:
   (i) requires care, treatment or control; and
   (ii) is incapable of managing himself or his affairs;
(b) is not under adequate care and control;
(c) is likely, by act or neglect, to cause death or serious bodily harm to himself or another person; and
(d) should in his own interest or in the public interest be taken into custody immediately ...

that medical practitioner or member of the Police Force may take that person into custody without a warrant.'[8]

Queensland 'On the grounds:

(a) that the patient is suffering from mental illness of a nature or to a degree that warrants the patient's detention in a hospital; and
(b) that the patient ought to be so detained in the interests of the patient's own welfare or with a view to the protection of other persons.'[9]

Appealing against compulsory treatment

Mental Health Review Boards or Tribunals in southern States, Western Australia and the Australian Capital Territory; the

Patient Review Tribunal in Queensland and the Supreme Court in the Northern Territory are able to review orders made under the relevant mental health act.

Police and transport to hospital

All jurisdictions permit police to enter premises, apprehend and transport people to hospital or other 'safe place'. In Victoria, guidelines state that we can request to be sedated to be transported, in which case an ambulance must be used.[10] If you're thinking clearly enough, you can use this to try to avoid the embarrassment of a trip in a divvy van.

Community treatment orders

In New South Wales, Victoria, Tasmania, the Australian Capital Territory and Western Australia, compulsory treatment outside of hospital can be ordered where the patient has refused treatment, subject to criteria similar or equivalent to those for compulsory treatment in hospital—that is, that the community treatment order is the 'least restrictive' alternative. Other jurisdictions can also make orders for community treatment. In New South Wales, a Community Counselling Order may also be made.

These Orders have the same effect as any other Court Order—there's a legal consequence if you breach the Order, including readmission to hospital. The Orders are usually given for a lengthy period of time (six to twelve months), depending on the statutory limit. They require the person to keep taking the prescribed medicine, for example, or stay at the same address.

Consent

Most jurisdictions specify that informed consent be gained prior to psychosurgery, electroconvulsive therapy (ECT), and non-psychiatric medical treatment. However, there are exceptions to this requirement. For example, in respect of ECT in Victoria: 'If your psychiatrist believes you are not able to give informed consent and ECT is necessary or if ECT is urgently needed, your psychiatrist can consent for you, even if you refuse.'[11] Although this only applies to people compulsorily admitted, a refusal or inability to consent to ECT could give your psychiatrist grounds to change your status from voluntary to compulsory and order ECT anyway.

The private system

Generally, mental health legislation does not apply to private psychiatric hospitals. Private hospitals may apply under the mental health legislation for a licence to operate or carry out electroconvulsive therapy.

Access to clinical files

Access to our own medical records is notoriously difficult to achieve. In some States, Freedom of Information legislation may be used to apply for access. Access to files held by private-sector practitioners and hospitals is more difficult; the courts have generally held that files on patients are the property of the practitioner or hospital who created them.

REMEDIES

The impotence of law

Most, if not all, of the mechanisms for complaint available to us are inaccessible, unenforceable, untimely, prohibitively expensive, lack independence, and/or provide no or inappropriate remedies. For instance, in Victoria with its apparently rights-based legislation, no patient has successfully sought to have a penalty imposed on a service provider.[12]

Operators of mainstream complaints avenues do not have particular expertise in mental health issues and thus may not fully comprehend the circumstances in which a complaint arose, nor the particular needs of a complainant. Equal opportunity legislation around the country is designed to mediate resolution of complaints, rather than establish legal precedent that changes laws.

Although complaints mechanisms are in place on paper, the fact that they are without effectiveness on the ground illustrates their tokenism. In practical terms, we have only unenforceable rights. Having said that, we still need to make complaints and challenge the system until we are heard.

Complaints against mental health services

You have the right to complain about any aspect of your hospital treatment, and equal opportunity law states that it's unlawful for you to be victimised if you do make a complaint. However, to be on the safe side, wait until you have been discharged (if possible) before you make a complaint. See Appendix III for complaints mechanisms.

Suing mental health services

Most of us are put off by the cost, time and stress involved in a civil action. However, people can get remarkably successful results by using the law. Frank sued a doctor who told him to cease taking lithium, resulting in a manic episode, from which he sustained many losses, including his job. Although Frank had to contend with many months of stress and stood to lose his home if he lost, he has sent a permanent, and effective, warning to psychiatrists on behalf of all of us.

Complaints against providers of goods and services

There are a large number of bodies established to resolve complaints and many of these are listed in Appendix III. Also, complaints can be made against individual professionals to their profession's governing body such as your State's Medical Board. Complaints can be made about quasi-judicial bodies through the Administrative Appeals Tribunal. Finding the best organisation to complain to is possibly the most important first step, and community legal centres or an advocacy organisation should be able to help.

OTHER LEGAL ISSUES

If you need to find out about the law relating to other issues such as family law, child protection, accommodation, crime and domestic violence, guides are available from the relevant government agencies and community legal centres, or if you have a social worker, you can request him or her to get information on your behalf.

Discrimination complaints

You might be able to make a complaint under your State's equal opportunity law or the Federal *Disability Discrimination Act* if you believe you've been treated unfairly because of your sex, disability, race, parental responsibilities, age or religion in any of the following areas:

- education;
- employment;
- accommodation;
- getting goods and using services;
- sport;
- land;
- access to public places;
- clubs and associations; or
- Commonwealth laws and programs.

Making a complaint involves putting your complaint in writing or, in some instances, being interviewed by one of the equal opportunity officers in your State capital. If this is in the 'too hard' basket when you're ill, you can put it off for up to twelve months. If the matter is urgent (for example being sacked because you've been ill), you can use an advocate, your trade union or a friend or family member to help.

All jurisdictions are required to try to resolve the complaint by conciliation. This can mean a meeting with the person you are complaining about with a member of the equal opportunity body being present so as to make sure everyone gets a fair say. This staff member is responsible for trying to get you and the other side to agree.

If you can't agree, you can generally take the matter to a hearing of the Board, Commission or Tribunal.

In many cases, an urgent or potential problem can be resolved within a few days. Other matters, however, have to wait in the queue—be prepared for a complaint to take months to be resolved. Nevertheless, it is still important to lodge a complaint. We don't get a fair go in many aspects of our lives, yet anti-discrimination laws are one of the few areas in which society is prepared to give us a fair go. On top of that, complaints create a cumulative effect on community awareness about our rights. By exercising our rights to use the law, we strengthen its impact; and bit by bit gradually change society so that other people experience a little less unfairness.

8

EMERGING FROM CRISIS

After a crisis or hospitalisation comes a phase of recovery. Still unwell, we find our lives in pieces and have to cope with many losses all at once. Not only that, the effects of medicine, whilst subduing troublesome symptoms, can affect our ability to think clearly and act decisively, and make it doubly difficult to resolve problems.

If you're reading this soon after a crisis, don't try to jump in and sort things out in a hurry. Recovery from illness can take a *long, long time*. And it's hard work.

Recovery is a time of grief as well. Give yourself the time and compassion to properly mourn the things you've lost. Make a list of the losses if you like. People have described to me their losses, and there's scarcely anything that is immune to the effects of manic depression:

LITANY OF LOSSES

Losses caused by the illness itself:

- identity;
- credibility;
- potency and capability to effect change and to rebuild;
- previous expectations;
- ability to do things as well as we used to;

- ability to relate optimally with our children, friends and partner;
- work satisfaction; and
- confidence.

Losses caused by the treatment:

- physical well-being (side-effects);
- libido;
- concentration, memory and alertness;
- self-esteem;
- identity as 'not-crazy';
- rights;
- independence;
- co-ordination; and
- creativity.

Possible losses within the family and the community

- partner/spouse;
- presence of children;
- capacity to exercise adult responsibility;
- job and/or career;
- income;
- accommodation;
- friends;
- ability to continue education;
- hobbies and sports;
- ability and right to manage own money;
- position in society; and
- hope.

Anyone who experienced more than one of these losses would be hard pressed to cope. So go easy on yourself and acknowledge the difficulty of the track ahead. Some strategies people use during the murky period after a crisis follow in the next section.

STRATEGIES

See yourself as 'well'

Trauma, or troubles of any sort, can shake a person's sense of who they are. A manic depression crisis can see us unravelling our identity and questioning our own and other people's values and beliefs about everything from the importance of work, education or money to the meaning of life itself. For many of us the questioning involves, for example religious or spiritual beliefs, on issues to do with suffering, mysticism and healing. Spiritual matters are discussed in Chapter 14 .

Expect to have to deal with some of these 'deep and meaningful' issues as a necessary part of your recovery, but remember you don't have to arrive at the answers tomorrow! This process can take years, and you'll discover that it's one of the positive outcomes of the suffering you're experiencing. You'll end up with a more considered approach to life and the world, and be more (*not* less) sure of yourself and your purpose. Take your time and enjoy the unfolding of new perspectives.

The first issue for many of us emerging from a crisis is coming to terms with being told, 'You've got a mental illness.' When we're first hospitalised, a typical reaction to fellow patients is, 'They're crazy, but not me.'

Eventually, however, we do recognise similarities between ourselves and others in hospital and we're challenged to redefine our self-image. The message is repeated over and over: 'You have a mental illness and you have to accept this as fact and take medicine for life.' Eventually the message takes effect as all good propaganda does and some of us conclude, '"They" must be right—I must be crazy.' Many of us revise our view of ourselves to that of 'nutters' or 'consumers' and give up on the idea of living a 'normal' life in the mainstream. Others absolutely refuse to accept the label. Most wrestle with the question for a long time.

When our identity as 'not-crazy' is challenged, we become

unsure of ourselves. So unsure that we might eventually give in to the pressure of the repeated, stigmatising message. We buy the false premise that being ‘crazy’ deserves loss of credibility and respectability. As we struggle with the unfairness of this, yet continue to punish ourselves with our new view of ourselves as ‘crazy’, we add ‘self-stigma’ to our list of problems.

We learn not to disclose our condition in case other people treat us unfairly. We learn to limit ourselves, redoubling our efforts to keep our expectations low.

Combatting self-stigma is difficult, especially if those around you keep reinforcing that you’re ill and/or incompetent. Maybe you *have* been ill, but it’s self-defeating to add to your own misery by believing you have no power to resume a normal life.

We do have the opportunity to take some control over manic depression. Though the condition has a biological basis, its relationship with triggers is not always consistent. The timing of episodes and our individual response to various medicines is not always predictable. But acknowledging these facts is not the same as saying, ‘I have no control over my condition.’ In fact, if we surrender control, others will take over for us. With apologies to St Francis[1]:

> *God, give me*
> *the gumption to take responsibility for rebuilding my life,*
> *the pragmatism to seek healing,*
> *and the faith to stay alive in the meantime.*

Taking control back is limited if you only look at your experiences through the ‘lifetime sentence’ perspective. There are alternative ways of thinking that allow for an optimistic outlook. ‘Mental illness’ is only one framework—one which carries somewhat pessimistic views about our capacity to have a fulfilling life. Perhaps you suffered a traumatic experience recently or in the far distant past—can you think of your current condition as a response to that trauma? Perhaps there's some spiritual learning to be done through your experiences with manic depression? Perhaps manic depression puts you among the elite of creative talent? Perhaps manic depression is a genetic variant that society needs for innovation, leadership and art?[2]

Look at your experiences in any way that makes sense to you. Just be sure that your perspective allows you to:

- accept that you have to deal with some problems, and
- never give up on yourself.

Never give up? Oh, dear, that's a tough one. Giving up is the sting in the tail of this mess, isn't it? The antidote is confidence. Pretend to be confident if you have to, and rescue your confidence after every setback. This involves taking a punt on yourself that you can carry something off. It might be small, such as phoning up to get information about a course at the community centre. Every time you do something you thought you couldn't, your confidence builds. Working with a counsellor on 'self-esteem' can also be useful.

It's often helpful to talk to other people who have manic depression, particularly those who have longer experience with it than you. If you don't know anyone, the Australian Mental Health Consumers' Network (see Appendix II) can put you in touch with your State delegate, who should be able to give you some local 'consumer-only' organisations to contact.

During your recovery, don't be tempted to cut off your links to your pre-illness aspirations. If you have long-term plans that you can't pursue now, put them on hold—don't scrap them in despair. Try and maintain as many contacts in the mainstream as you can. By 'mainstream' I mean ordinary activities that have nothing whatsoever to do with mental health, for example participating in your usual sport, keeping up with friends who don't have a mental illness, continuing your involvement in your child's school. Take a leave of absence from mainstream activities if you need to, but plan on returning as soon as you can.

If you've lost all your mainstream contacts and activities, as many of us do, start with something interesting and easy to break into. Read something other than self-help books! Look up old friends who don't have a mental illness, or sign up for a short course offered by a mainstream organisation where you'll meet other people who aren't necessarily 'consumers'. The noticeboards at libraries and community centres often have local activities that might interest you. If you go to a disability support centre, ask the staff to help you get back into the mainstream (it's their job, actually!). Get back into the workforce, even if it's only casual work for an hour a week. Your views of yourself and what might be possible will change when you are among people whose lives don't revolve around mental illness.

This is not to say you should desert the mental health enclave. We draw strength and learn from friends who have similar experiences; our recovery is assisted by the positive offerings of psychiatry. It's comfortable and legitimate to be among people who don't get upset if you're unwell. Among others with manic depression and other mental illnesses, you'll find people who want to fight the injustices of how we're treated by society. So use the enclave to gather strength between forays into the mainstream.

If an episode of manic depression returns, it is absolutely normal and appropriate to be disappointed and angry. Often this starts the whole process of recovery. But you will have learned from the previous episode a little of what to expect. If you have a sense of 'Here we go again', you're close to being able to draw on your experience, so you can plan to prevent the next episode and limit its potential damage. The next chapter gives steps you can follow after you've recovered to plan for the future.

In summary:

- expect to have to address fundamental questions about yourself, life and the world;
- identify the ways you view having manic depression;
- consider the effects of 'self-stigma';
- talk to other people with manic depression or other mental illnesses;
- don't scrap long-term plans—put them on hold until you can revise them properly;
- don't give up on resuming life in the mainstream; and
- expect to be angry or disappointed if you have another episode.

How to get moving

The sheer number and complexity of problems to deal with can be enough to drive you to drink or under the bedclothes. Don't panic! Have a drink or a sleep *after* you've done this exercise devised by the ten-year-old child of a woman with manic depression.[3] Do it now—you can always read the rest of this later.

Think of the emperor penguins in Antarctica. They all huddle in a group to keep warm, shuffling around in a spiral so they can all take turns in being on the cold outside and then warm themselves up on the inside of the group. The coldest penguins on the outside of the circle are equivalent to the most pressing or important issues that need to be dealt with. The penguins on the inside are warm, so they can wait for your attention.

Now, your penguins can keep shuffling around forever, but if you leave them to their shuffling, the same penguins will keep getting cold in their turn, *ad infinitum*. Similarly, if you leave issues unaddressed, they'll keep popping up for attention.

1. Draw a circle representing the mass of penguins. On the outside of the circle, list the most pressing of issues for today or this week. On the inside, list any issues that aren't

of *immediate* concern. Once you've identified the coldest 'penguins', write down for each of them:

- what you want to achieve that will solve the problem;
- the first step towards solving the problem.

2. Then carry out those first steps. If there are phone calls or appointments to be made, make them now or at the next opportunity.

3. At your leisure, consider and write out all the steps you'll need to take to deal with the coldest penguins.

As you progressively work on warming up the coldest penguins, you can start to look at others with less pressing needs.

This exercise often highlights the need for know-how and advice from other people, and sometimes some practical help. Don't be afraid to ask people you trust to help.

When you're wading through the priority issues, don't be tempted to look back too often for evidence that you're getting on top of things. If you try to compare this week with last week, you'll be disappointed if you see no progress—and despair or panic if things seem worse this week. Measure your progress only once every six to twelve months, and you will see improvements in some areas of your life.

One of the traps of rebuilding from serious disaster is the tendency to forget to do things for fun, or to put off recreation because it doesn't seem to be a top priority. Sometimes the fun is elusive, especially when the tail end of depression seemingly hangs around forever. Still, promise yourself one or two treats a week. Treats don't have to be complicated or expensive—take some enjoyment from having a coffee with a friend, walking in a park, or bookshop-browsing.

In summary:

- act on top priorities only—the 'coldest penguins';
- use supportive counselling or practical help from others;

- don't look back too often; and
- put some fun back.

Overcoming barriers created by medicine

In the period following a crisis, barriers to getting moving can be compounded by the unwanted effects of medicine. Going to work when your concentration is lousy is damned near impossible. Getting your relationship back together would be hard enough but when the medicine makes you impotent, ruins your sex drive or stops you from achieving orgasm, it's tough on both partners.

There's little you can do to directly overcome these barriers, especially if you can't switch medicines or lower the dose of the medicinal culprits. Grieve for what has been lost and hope that it's only temporary. In the meantime, report the unwanted effects and request that the medicine(s) be changed.

If your job allows, use your diary, a notebook or a whiteboard to keep work priorities in mind. Plan each day's tasks so you intersperse 'thinking' work with work that doesn't require much concentration. Try to schedule meetings for the time of day when you're at your most lucid. See Chapter 10 for other strategies for employment.

Some people find they can no longer play their favourite sport or musical instrument because of lithium's unwanted effects. This can be devastating, but is likely to be viewed as a trivial complaint by mental health workers unless you're an Olympian or a virtuoso. If you can't reduce or switch medicines, your next best option may be to find an alternative way of enjoying sport or music.

At home, keep the lines of communication open. If medicine is causing problems with sex, report the fact to your psychiatrist and see if you can switch medicine or lower the dose. Talk about it with your partner; you may decide together it's better to settle for cuddles for a while. If your partner is willing, go together to a mainstream counsellor, or go alone for ideas about things that you can do to improve things. There are other ideas about relationships in Chapter 12.

If sedation is a problem, get help with household chores from wherever you can find it, so you can devote the little energy you have to being available to your children. Do as much as you can with the children and accept non-threatening help. Chapter 13 gives other ideas for parenting with manic depression.

Coping with a community treatment order

If you're on a community treatment order, don't waste energy getting cross about something you can't change immediately. Play the game for the duration and use the period of the order to develop your own plans for controlling your condition. Rebuild your mental health workers' trust in you. Basically, you're on the order because they don't believe you'll take their prescribed medicine. You have to work on demonstrating they can trust you to manage your condition. So take the stuff, and use your visits to demonstrate your commitment to resuming your normal life. Ask them what they can do to help; ask them what else they recommend you do in addition to taking medicine; ask them if they have any reading matter that might help. Then follow up on what they suggest. If they have no suggestions apart from taking medicine, use the ideas in this book to do it yourself, and make sure you let them know how conscientiously you're working on your recovery.

If your order has to be reviewed by a board or tribunal, prepare for the hearing. Get information from the mental health worker, or the board or tribunal, about the hearing itself. If there's a mental health law service in your State, ask them to help you prepare. You might get an independent opinion from another psychiatrist. Organise an advocate, lawyer or friend to attend the hearing with you. Apply for a copy of your medical records so you can discover what the 'other side' think about you, and be prepared to counter their likely arguments.

You might find you have to tackle some other issues that work against your credibility in the eyes of the board or tribunal. If you take action on issues such as illicit drug and alcohol overuse, you'll get extra 'brownie points' at the hearing (and you'll probably be healthier too!). If, during the period of the order, you've managed to resolve some critical social issues like dealing with a toxic relationship or organising stable accommodation, this too will add to your chances of getting off the order.

If you want the maximum degree of control over your manic depression and your life, you have to arrange things so that the mental health laws don't get an opportunity to take that control away from you. There are a number of things you can do to achieve this. One is to seek referral from the mental health service to a private psychiatrist; another is to get private health insurance so if you need hospitalisation you can get in before you've totally 'lost it'—well before the mental health system decides you need compulsory treatment. You can establish your own emergency team—choose willing people from trusted friends or family members, a general practitioner, your pharmacist, your psychiatrist, psychologist or counsellor. The most important step, though, is to build your credibility by actively managing your manic depression. (See next chapter.)

Longer term rebuilding

As you progressively solve the priority problems, you can start to use a more focussed approach to planning. If you have a favourite technique for planning, use it, or adapt a system from other self-help books. You can keep using the 'cold penguins' approach if you like.

Visualise how life will be when you've achieved what you want. To make sure you don't miss any important aspect of life, draw for yourself a 'wheel' like the one opposite.

Pick from the wheel a small number of long-term goals. Write the goals down, being as specific as you can. Consider how long each goal might take to realise. List the milestones you think you'll reach along the way. Under each milestone, list:

1. The individual tasks you'll need to carry out to reach the milestone;
2. The barriers you expect to encounter; and
3. Sources of information, guidance or help you can call on.[4]

Start the first task, then do the next one and the next. Review your progress at each milestone, or when you get stuck. Give yourself time off from the plan when you need to; go easy on yourself when new barriers crop up. Good luck!

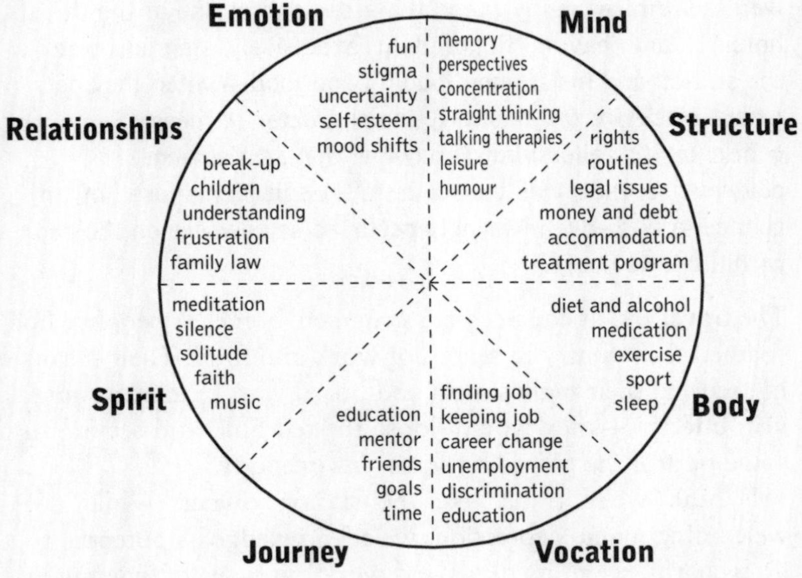

Figure 8.2 Planning wheel

9

THE ART OF ROLLER-COASTER RIDING

At the station where I worked [in the Victorian Wimmera district] for some time as a 'knock-about man', three cooks were kept during the 'wallaby' season—one for the house, one for the men, and one for the travellers. Moreover, 'travellers' would not infrequently spend the afternoon at one of the three hotels ... and, having 'liquored up' extensively, stagger up to the station and insist upon lodging and food—which they got. I have no desire to take away the character of these gentlemen travellers; but I may mention as a strange coincidence, that, was the requested hospitality refused by any chance, a bush-fire invariably occurred somewhere on the run within twelve hours.[1]

The travellers, of course, were swagmen, homeless people who roamed the country in search of work and food. Their means of securing their night's meal and board was, on this account, very effective—they would 'loose the red bull' and set fire to some part of the offending squatter's property.

I think we're a bit like the station owner. While not welcoming manic depression, we acknowledge its potential to do us harm, see to its needs and work out ways of living with it. When we do that, we can turn our attention to the most important challenge of all: to lead a full life.

STEP 1—TELLING THE DIFFERENCE BETWEEN ILLNESS AND A BAD DAY

I am indebted to my friend Bernie[2] for his common-sense approach to life on the roller-coaster. He keeps a list like the one below on his fridge and before he allows himself to consider the possibility that he is getting sick, he excludes all the usual reasons why people feel lousy. Here's my interpretation of his list—you can create your own.

I'm probably just having a bad day if some of these apply…

- I've had more or less coffee today than usual
- I've had more or less alcohol today than usual
- I've had more or less tobacco today than usual
- I've not had enough sex or too much bad sex lately
- I've spoken to my mother/ex/other *agent provocateur* today
- My period is due soon
- It's a full moon
- It's been extremely hot
- I've done more or less exercise than usual today/lately
- My face has erupted in pimples
- I have another illness or aches and pains today
- I've been inside all day
- My car broke down
- Work was particularly stressful today
- I ignored my dog/cat/goldfish today
- I haven't played nor listened to music today
- I haven't eaten as well as usual today
- I'm cross about something
- I'm worried about money
- I'm worried about getting too fat
- I've got too much to do
- I haven't got enough to do
- My kid is sick or cranky.

STEP 2—USING MOOD, ACTIVITY AND THINKING TO IDENTIFY SIGNPOSTS

If we're going to find useful, practical and reliable guides to our condition, we can't rely on the lists of symptoms that usually accompany the 'wavy line' model (see Chapter 3). Watching out for general 'hyperactivity' can't be a reliable indicator—we might just be particularly busy for a while. Neither is watching for 'elation' or 'despair' reliable as these are normal human emotions.

Some people use questionnaires like the Beck Depression Inventory[3] or the Altman Self-Rating Mania Scale.[4] While they're useful to keep track of our overall well-being, they don't help us work out what to do to prevent damage.

How to identify your own signposts

Figure 9.1 shows some general descriptions of the different 'symptoms' of manic depression.

The problem with these general descriptions is that they aren't specific to individual people and are not very useful as signals of oncoming illness.

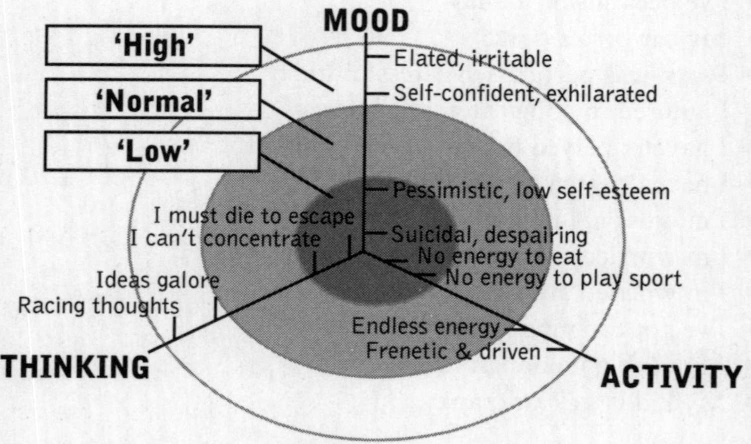

Figure 9.1 Some typical—but not necessarily personal—descriptions of changes during mood disturbance

We need to get more specific about the circumstances that tell us reliably whether we're 'going off'. If we search for our own typical experiences of changes, we can develop our own set of warning signs. To be useful, these changes have to be

- typical for us when we're unwell or becoming unwell;
- unusual for us when we're well; and
- concrete and specific.

As a rule of thumb, these typical changes are more reliable indicators of illness when they involve changes in mood, activity and thinking, but there are exceptions—sometimes a single event can be a useful tip-off. I discovered, for example, that if I can't decide *whether* I want to buy anything for lunch (let alone *choose* something to buy), it's more than likely I'm becoming depressed, even if I don't feel lousy. In this instance the thinking, not the mood feeling, is the thing that tips me off that a mood shift could be happening.

Rachel, for example, notices the number of lay-by dockets in her purse mounting and knows she's moving towards mania. For Carole, Mary, Greg, Marilyn, Wendy and Jonathan the most reliable signpost is sleep loss at the onset of a high episode. Wendy has another signpost: she is told she 'talks too much' during hypomania. Shane only plays the piano when he's hypomanic, and he does this often enough during hypomania for it to be a useful signpost.

Figure 9.2 is an illustration of some of the typical personal signposts people have told me they look out for.

There seems to be a different set of patterns, or signposts, for the beginning of a mood disturbance and another set when the disturbance has become severe. The Early Warning signposts are like small amber coloured road signs. This is the time to put on the brakes.

The signposts of more severe illness are like large, red road signs. They tell us that we are in danger of sustaining losses and tell us to jump for our safety nets.

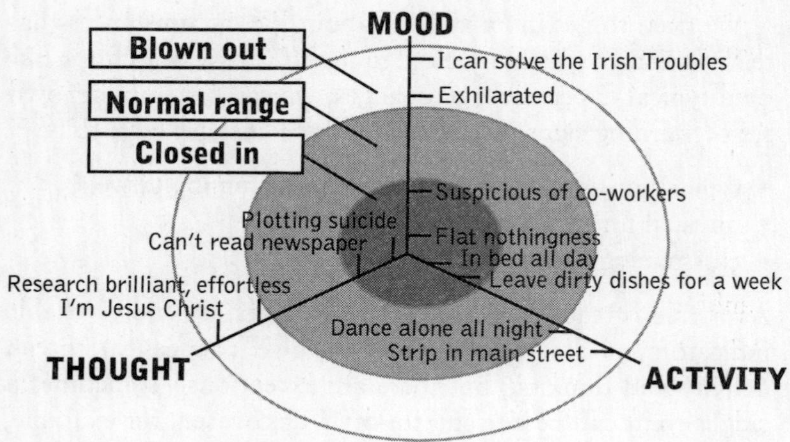

Figure 9.2 Some aggregated personal experiences of individuals

These days, I know that if I'm thinking about working for an escort agency then I'm usually severely unwell—more than I realise at the time. Wendy says if she's dressing in sexually provocative clothes, she knows she's very ill. She tries to intervene before this stage, before she loses too much perspective.

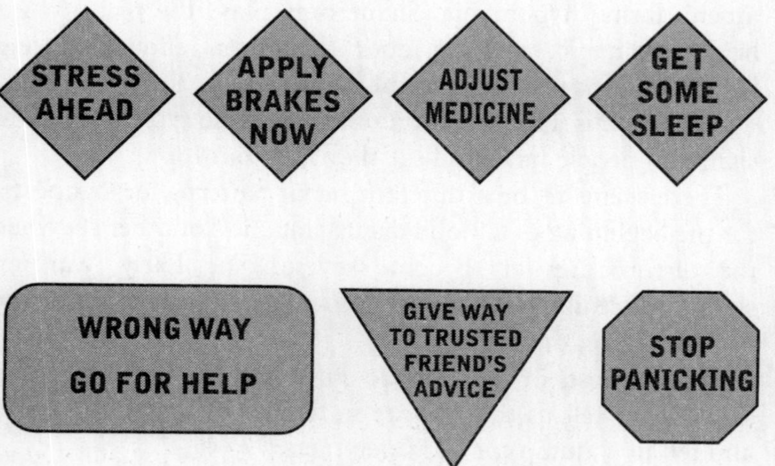

Luckily, for most people the speed of onset of an episode is roughly the same from episode to episode. Some, like me, have a fairly slow build-up, over weeks or months, so I can put on the brakes in the early stages. Others find a major episode can ambush them suddenly—as quickly as overnight. If your episodes happen suddenly, you'll need to rely more on safety nets because you might not have time to jump on the brakes.

To start off, simply keep a record of your mood, activity and thinking over a period of time—say three months. Look for changes in:

- mood—optimistic or a pessimistic view of the world; irritability, grandiosity or nothingness
- activity—unusually high or low levels of activity, or exaggerated or 'weird' activity
- thinking—the contents of the thoughts, or the thinking process, for example thought contents might express a death wish. Thought processes might demonstrate 'off' judgment or decision-making.

You can make a note of mood/activity/thinking as it occurs, or you can work from experience of previous episodes. Another source I used was my journal. Go at a sustainable pace.

> *Caution: When we're not well, we dismiss things as being too much effort, or trivial, or too complex, or not worth doing. If you're feeling like this now, don't try the exercises that follow. These exercises rely on having adequate mental and emotional resources and a sense that your perspective and judgment are reasonably sound. If you're ill, your time might be better spent recovering, resting, taking things at your own pace and leaving this exercise until you're well again.*

Write the mood, activity or thinking down in five or six words—just enough to identify it in your mind. See Table 9.1.

In the next column, identify whether the behaviour you've

noticed is primarily a mood, an activity or a thinking process. Try listing some more behaviours so you have a good selection of moods, activities and thinking.

Which way does the sign point? Next, for each mood, activity, thought or thinking process, assign a direction to the signpost:

- ▲—high, hypomanic, manic, blown out;
- ▼—blue, depressed, suicidal, closed in;
- ▲▼—all over the place, fast mood swings, relevant to both depression and mania (useful as a signal that 'something' is going on).

Try listing some more behaviours so you have a good selection of the directions that are most relevant to you.

How to tell if a signpost is reliable Work out the reliability of each signpost. Make an estimate of how often this mood, activity, thought or thinking process has happened when you have been ill. Has it only happened during one episode? Does it happen every time you go off?

The most useful signpost behaviours are those that happen 'often when sick, rarely when well'. Give these a number 'I' rating on the chart.

I	often	rarely
sick	x	
well		x

Of lesser value are those which happen 'often when sick and often when well' and 'rarely when sick and rarely when well'. This sort of signpost rates a 'II' or 'III' on the chart. With a bit of common sense, some of these behaviour patterns can become useful backup signposts.

For example, I yell at my child from time to time whether I

am sick or well. But there is an important qualitative difference in what I say to my child, how I say it and my child's response. I have learned that if there is fear in his face, I am looking at a signpost.

If there are any moods, activities or thinking that could be normal for you in certain contexts (for example 'Writing business plan for new business') describe the context in which it's an indicator. (See Table 9.1).

II	often	rarely
sick	x	
well	x	

or

III	often	rarely
sick		x
well		x

The moods, activities and thinking that can never qualify as signposts are those that occur 'rarely when sick, often when well.'

If you haven't got many signposts with a reliability rating of I, try to identify some more over a longer period of time. It took me months before the penny dropped that my difficulty with deciding what to have for lunch was a signpost!

Early warning or major alert? Indicate whether the sign is typically an early or late one in the course of your condition. For example, when I wake up to a feeling of dread, I'm usually still working, and so am not yet hospital material. I'd call this an early warning. When Rachel discovers a purse full of lay-bys, she usually ends up in hospital within weeks. She would call this a major alert.

If you can't find any obvious early warning signs, take some more time and consider carefully the events in the days, weeks and months leading up to an episode.

Your final list might look like Table 9.1. If you prefer a picture to a list, you can draw your own version of Figure 9.2.

Signpost-spotting with a friend

This technique is effective when you do it on your own, but it can be helpful if someone who knows you very well and whom you trust also helps you spot signposts. Before you ask someone to help, consider this caution:

> CAUTION
>
> *Worried carers can sometimes overreact to the appearance of a signpost and it's important to remember that a single swallow doesn't make a summer.*
>
> *No relationship can afford to have these signposts turned from useful tools into lists of prohibited activities.*

To avoid this possibility, discuss it with your friend and decide whether you want their help. Equally, be prepared for your friend to decline your invitation—they might be afraid of being blamed for 'taking over' from you or they might be unable to cope with the extra responsibility you're asking them to take on.

Hints for friends helping hunt signposts Identifying changes in activity is fairly straightforward, but because thinking and mood are internal, subjective elements, your friend will have to rely on outward signs, acting with the objectivity of a scientific observer.

Your friend can identify changes in mood by the subjects you talk about and non-verbal clues such as crying and posture. How you generally look can also indicate your mood—a 'depressed face', tired, with heavy lids can be a give-away sign of a depressed mood to an experienced observer.

To get an idea of whether your thinking is 'off', your friend will need to rely on the subject and pace of your speech and whether your judgment appears to be different from usual.

Useful signposts for me				
Description (5 or 6 words only)	**M, A or T**	**Direction**	**Reliability**	**Early warning? Major alert?**
Waking up feeling nothingness	M	↓	I	Early warning (depression)
Not returning phone calls or answering the phone	A	↓	I	Early warning (depression)
Having afternoon naps	A	↓	II	Early warning (depression) if combined with boredom
Can't decide what to have for lunch	T	↓	I	Early warning (depression)
Cranky and critical at work	M	↑↓	II	Early warning (non-specific)
Yelling at kids	A	↑↓	II	Early warning (non-specific) if kids react in fear
Can't settle to watch TV	A	↑	I	Early warning (hypomania)
Life of the party, inventing new words, hilarious	A	↑	I	Early warning (hypomania) if others are telling me to shut up

Table 9.1 Examples of signposts

Useful signposts for me				
Description (5 or 6 words only)	**M, A or T**	**Direction**	**Reliability**	**Early warning? Major alert?**
Writing a business plan for new business	A	▲	II	Early warning (mania) if it's a brand new idea and other early warning signs are present
Ringing friends and talking for hours	A	▲	I	Early warning (mania)
Long philosophical discussions	T	▲	II	Early warning (black mania) if I'm angry and planning political revolt, and if combined with sleep loss and drinking
Having trouble speaking and moving	A	▼	I	Major alert (depression)
People at work out to get me	T	▼	I	Major alert (depression)
Going to church and being overwhelmed by the beauty and the presence of God	M	▲	III	Major alert (mania) only if combined with other signposts

Table 9.1 cont Examples of signposts

Useful signposts for me				
Description (5 or 6 words only)	**M, A or T**	**Direction**	**Reliability**	**Early warning? Major alert?**
Out all night drinking in Kings Cross	A	↑	I	Major alert (mania)
Getting into fights	A	↑	I	Major alert (mania)
Buying stuff I wouldn't ordinarily want, using credit cards	A	↑	I	Major alert (mania)
Seeing the answer to a complex political problem	T	↑	II	Major alert (mania) but only if I'm not a politician yet I'm planning to go to Canberra today to tell the prime minister

Table 9.1 cont Examples of signposts

Using the approach described over, your friend can compile their own list of signposts.

Compare the two lists. Clarify any items on your friend's list that are uncomfortable or surprising. Discuss whether you agree about the signposts' reliability and status as early warnings or major alerts. Compile a joint list (see example in Table 9.2) or draw a picture based on Figure 9.2.

STEP 3—CREATING BRAKES AND SAFETY NETS

I don't like standing near the edge of a platform when an express train is passing through. I like to stand right back and if possible to get a pillar between me and the train.

Winston Churchill[5]

And Levin, a happy father and a man in perfect health, was several times so near suicide that he hid the cord, lest he be tempted to hang himself, and was afraid to go out with his gun, for fear of shooting himself.

Leo Tolstoy, Anna Karenina

Early warning signposts—put on the brakes

Especially in the early stages, we can influence our condition by using Brakes we've planned in advance.

Some brakes that people use include:

- increasing the dose of certain medicines as agreed with the psychiatrist;
- having some reiki or other healing;
- staying away from conversations, environments or activities that rev them up;
- making a list of things to do for the day and not doing anything not on the list;
- using up excess energy with sport, chopping wood, housework;

Some changes I notice when my friend is ill				
Description (5 or 6 words only)	**M, A or T**	**Direction**	**Reliability**	**Early warning? Major alert?**
Eyes are 'switched off'	M	↓	I	Major alert
Rings many friends and talks for hours	A	↑	I	Early warning
Buys stuff she wouldn't ordinarily want	A	↑	I	Major alert
Stays out all night drinking	A	↑	I	Major alert
Looks dishevelled	M	↓	II	Major alert
Speaks slowly with lots of pauses	T	↓	I	Major alert
Puts self down	M	↓	I	Early warning

Table 9.2 Sample observations by a trusted friend

- taking time off work; and
- calling the psychiatrist.

If a friend is participating, discuss your expectations of each other. You might decide that your friend will, on noticing one or more signposts, simply let you know and leave the rest up to you. This could be as simple as accepting your need to withdraw from a conversation that is revving you up too much. Try, as long as your condition permits, to keep the control in your own hands. Carers are much more likely to stand back, however nervously, if they see us actively taking steps to manage our illness.

Other people can be approached to help us put the brakes on. For example, because Greg can't take lithium for medical reasons he totally relies on signs. He knows from experience that for him, mania comes first and it isn't always followed by depression. He also knows that large doses of chlorpromazine (Largactil®) will stop a manic episode dead in its tracks. Greg has made arrangements with his psychiatrist and his general practitioner to be prepared to prescribe him sufficient chlorpromazine when *he* says he needs it.

If the brakes fail, we can rely on safety nets if we've put them in place.

Major alert signposts—rely on your safety nets

If you're confronted by a big, red signpost, chances are you're already sick and may become very sick. This is when your safety nets come into play. Their most important function is to make sure you stay alive.

The most important safety net is to listen to your trusted friend or your mental health professionals. You may also have arranged that your friend will step in if your judgment slips away without you noticing.

Frank finds that there's a very short time before his mania ambushes him, leaving only hours from the start of symptoms to being totally out of touch with reality. In Frank's case, safety nets are more important than brakes. Apart from deciding to stay on lithium, Frank has arranged safety nets that are constantly ready to catch him. He has arranged access to an emergency supply of lithium from the pharmacy and for more than one doctor to be familiar with the track record of his illness.

Some other ideas are:

- educate your family so they can stop worrying and start getting involved in supporting your efforts to manage your illness;
- keep up your health insurance if you prefer private hospitals and can afford it;
- get an after-hours emergency phone number for your psychiatrist or mental health team; and
- persuade your mental health team to give you more intensive support when you say you need it. (Difficult but not impossible!)

Safety nets and other strategies for education, work, money, relationships, children and spiritual issues are included in later chapters.

Safety nets, brakes and suicide

Life is sweet perhaps to some, but I prefer what is sweeter than life, and that is death. So goodbye forever, my dear parents. It is nobody's fault, but a strong desire of my own which I have longed to fulfill for three or four years. I have always had a hope that some day I might have all opportunity of fulfilling it, and now it has come... It is a wonder I have put this off so long, but I thought perhaps I should cheer up a bit and put all thought out of my head...I know there is no forgiveness for what I am going to do. I am tired of living, so am willing to die. Life may be sweet to some, but death to me is sweeter.[6]

I can remember talking to him and he was saying 'I don't know why I want to kill myself. You know the thing that keeps you alive? Well, something else is pulling me in the other direction. I just can't stop it.'

Jane

'Yet,' says Tolstoy, 'whilst my intellect was working, something else in me was working too, and kept me from the deed—consciousness of life, as I may call it ...'[7]

Rachel didn't believe she could possibly survive more than a handful of years.

In my life, I didn't think I'd be older than Marilyn Monroe, but I am. Once upon a time if somebody said to me 'You're going to reach 38 years of age', I would have laughed at them. I would have said 'I know how to stop that.' Even though I say something like that, I've never ever tried to kill myself ... and just the thought of it—I could never—I'm too gutless for that. I am.

Brakes A well-experienced depressive friend of mine has had plenty of opportunities to reflect on suicide. He realised that, as he did for other unwanted thoughts, he could disengage from thoughts of killing himself.

> *Just because you think of doing something doesn't mean you have to do it!*

With practice, we can separate from suicidal thoughts, becoming a disinterested observer. The trick is not to let the thoughts create so much panic that you can't 'hear' alternative thoughts such as 'This will pass'.

This is particularly useful in non-crisis situations. Sometimes we can be bothered for weeks or months by vague, low-impact suicidal thoughts that aren't accompanied by a burning desire or a plan to carry out the act. As Tolstoy observed: 'During the whole course of this year ... when I almost unceasingly kept asking myself how to end the business, whether by the rope or by the bullet.'[8]

Keep your trusted friend and mental health team up to date about the thoughts in case they start to escalate.

If you're resolved to kill yourself, delay as long as possible before taking steps of actually doing it. Keep yourself alive until the compulsion wanes—as it will, eventually, with or without medicine.

Sometimes, despite our efforts, we know the brakes are failing. When you can't keep the thoughts at arms length any more, or you start to be swept into carrying out a suicide attempt, jump for your safety net.

Safety nets The most important safety net when you're feeling suicidal—being rescued by a trusted friend or mental health professional—has a major downfall: you might have to activate it yourself by telling someone what you need. You may have occasional flashes of wanting to initiate your rescue. Strike while the iron's hot and act on these flashes.

Get on the phone and call your emergency team, psychiatrist, anyone. Send the mayday. Get hold of that trusted friend and see if he or she can come over for a while. If you're agitated and you've agreed with your psychiatrist that you can take additional doses of medicine, take some. Obviously, don't overdose!

Last, while you're waiting for the crisis to subside, be patient. This will pass, but only if you stay alive. Try to believe it.

STEP 4—STRATEGIES FOR STAYING WELL

If you stay well in mind, body and spirit, manic depression is less likely to hit. And if it does hit again, it will cause less damage if you are already generally healthy.

Here are some of the steps that can be taken to limit recurrences of manic depression and their consequences:

- get regular sleep;
- eat a moderate, balanced diet;
- stop drinking to kill the pain/restlessness/isolation;
- pay attention to your physical health and seek treatment from medical and alternative therapists;
- get enough exercise;
- get involved in important issues, jobs or your personal vision;
- pay attention to the spiritual dimension if it is relevant to you; and
- get into some mainstream activities.

STEP 5—LET TIME DO ITS WORK

The important thing to remember is that time is an important ingredient in successfully managing manic depression. We need to be well enough to tune in to our own experience with manic depression. Over time, we get better at noticing early signs. Putting on the brakes effectively takes practice; safety nets take time to set up. Take it easy. Let the passing of time teach you your recovery.

10

HOW TO GET YOUR FOOT IN THE DOOR—AND STAY INSIDE

In this chapter we'll consider how manic depression disrupts our education and employment, and the ways of limiting the damage. Manic depression can start at any age and for many people, that means teenage years. Although this chapter focuses on managing tertiary education and employment, many of the strategies can be used by people in their teens.

THE GETTING OF WISDOM

Remember Jonathan's story of failing in the odd years of his university degree, while romping in with distinctions in the even years? Rachel was training as a teacher when illness struck; I was in medical school; Kate was studying to be an engineer.

When manic depression threatens your education, there are a number of strategies you can use to limit the damage.

Disability services

Most tertiary institutions have a disability services unit which can help individual students on request. Although it can be difficult to see yourself as 'having a disability' and you need to disclose your condition, these services can be helpful if the going gets tough. They can help with admissions, appeals, access, varied study and attendance arrangements, and leave of absence.

Many courses reserve a number of places for people with a disability and you can find out about these from the admissions office or the disability unit on campus.

If you think you're not getting a fair go (for example not being allowed an extension, not being allowed to sit a supplementary exam, not being allowed in to a particular subject) and it's to do with your illness or the fact that you've been unwell in the past or might become unwell again, see the people at the disability unit on campus, as they may be able to help you by intervening informally or with a formal complaint.

If the disability unit can't help, you might have to take the matter through the institution's grievance procedure on your own. Going it alone, especially when we're recovering from illness, is a high-risk, high-distress strategy. Get someone to advocate for you and help with the red tape. This could be a fellow student or the Student Union might be able to give some assistance. Your State anti-discrimination or equal opportunity commission can also give advice and if the matter falls under their jurisdiction they will also receive, investigate and mediate a complaint.

Stay enrolled as long as you can

When we're ill, we don't always make sound judgments. Try to avoid making any major decision—including whether to drop out of your course—until you're well again. Take leave of absence if you need more time to recover, because chances are that in a year you'll be back in the pink. As Jan Stumbles puts it, 'The only thing left is to grit your teeth and wait. Try and wait it out.'[1]

If you're faced with the choice between dropping out or asking for special consideration, don't cut off your nose to spite your face. If you ask for special consideration and have to tell the institution the reason, you run the risk of your credibility being diminished and possibly damaging your eventual professional reputation. If you drop out, you won't have a profession, let alone a professional reputation to protect.

So, start with a trustworthy teacher, or someone at the disability unit on campus. Let him or her know:

- what might or is likely to happen in class and with your assignments if you get sick;
- what action you will take in the event of becoming ill; and
- what you want from the teacher.

You could ask for approval-in-principle for submitting late assignments. Teachers might be hesitant to give you *carte blanche*, but raising the possibility at the beginning of the year paves the way for a request if winter blues or exam-season mania hit. You could ask the teacher to advocate for you, if necessary, in any dealings with the course administration and other teachers.

If you're hospitalised for a lengthy period, have any important and urgent school work brought to the hospital once you have recovered sufficiently to be able to study. Classmates can help by collecting handouts from classes you miss, and especially in a small study group, by helping each other understand key concepts and pooling resources for research.

Don't worry about having to drop out

If you've already taken as much time off as they'll allow and now have no choice but to drop out, don't allow yourself to stress about how disastrous it feels. Have another look at Rational Emotive Therapy (Chapter 5). People around you might be tut-tutting and saying, 'What a pity you won't become a …' This is not helpful talk. Ignore it. Focus on recovery and have a look at alternative careers that might actually suit you better anyway.

CAREER CHOICES AND CHANGING TACK

Every time I got sick I used to try to rebuild my life in the same way. It's like my life is a wine glass—when I get sick, it would get smashed. So I'd try and put it back together the same way. Each time it got smashed, it became harder and harder to get it back into the right shape. One day I realised that it was useless to try to make another wine glass. I used the bits of glass to make a tiger ... I was never supposed to be a wine glass in the first place!

Anon[2]

Career choices are made according to lots of criteria, some conscious, others hidden. When I was eighteen, I changed my preferences after getting better marks than expected—I decided I would follow my father into medicine. When I was 27, I took a year off work and set up my own secretarial agency. When I was 36, I decided to devote more time to writing, in the pursuit of a career that would meet my needs for recognition, solitude and intellectual challenge.

One of the best things about having manic depression is the capacity for reflection and courage to embark on change that it brings. Be guided by your common sense or your gut instincts—whichever is most reliable for you. Take advice from trusted and qualified career advisors. Make use of all the disability services you can—you deserve them. Ask yourself the following questions:

What am I good at? What do I like? Luckily, 'doing what we like' is often the same as 'doing what we're good at'.

You can get an idea of your preferred work style using the Myers-Briggs Type Indicator™ from any of a number of popular books. The Type Indicator looks at four key questions:

1. Where do I like to focus my attention? (extroversion/introversion);
2. How do I acquire information? (sensing/intuition);

3. How do I make decisions? (thinking/feeling); and
4. How do I like to deal with the outside world? (judging/perceiving).[3]

What do others I respect think? In the hands of a good vocational counsellor our preferences for which skills we use and what we're seeking in a job/career become starkly clear. A vocational counsellor is usually a qualified psychologist who will interview you to see how you tick and take into account your history with illness. A number of psychological tests add to the information from the interview and enable the vocational counsellor to give often surprising suggestions.

My vocational counsellor pointed out that I'd been moving to more and more creative roles. The combined results of a series of pyschometric tests revealed that my preferences were for creative jobs.

I whispered to her, 'Does this mean I can be a writer?'

Of course, I didn't need her permission, only my own. I might never make any money out of writing, but to 're-frame' myself as a writer instantly brought me the confidence I needed.

Many of us have a creative stripe that seems to come with the manic-depressive territory, and we can add this to our melting pot of options in careers and/or retraining.

You can get the perspectives of friends, colleagues and professionals whom you trust to tell you accurately and constructively what they have observed of you in your work and other roles. However, be aware that they will hold different perspectives. The opinions of family members are often limited by their experience of our illness, so they may not share your positive outlook.

Most psychiatrists encourage people to return to work. However, they stay in business by being conservative. If you want to borrow a million dollars to set up a 'Jurassic Park' in far north-west Western Australia, don't be surprised if your shrink thinks you might be getting manic. On the other hand, if this is your dream of a lifetime and you have the skills and connections to carry it off, it's important to pursue it.

How can we tell if conservative advice is restrictive for the sake of being restrictive or is actually in our best interests? We have to listen primarily to ourselves. Is there a whooshing sound of escalating mania in the background? Is there a creepy feel of paranoia? Or can you honestly say there is neither? Can you rationally counter most or all the arguments against your plans? Have you thought about safety nets in case you become ill again? Can the career plan survive a mood shift?

Will my plans make me enough money? Making enough money for survival or prosperity is a criterion that goes without saying, but defining what is *enough* depends on your goals and how much you are prepared to adapt your lifestyle. It's not easy to learn to live on less, but it's certainly not impossible, and sometimes unexpected benefits, such as less stress, a healthier diet, more exercise and discovery of resourcefulness, can flow from living on a lower income.

Set your goals for career/job and lifestyle. Then factor in the likelihood and possible cost of future illness and work out how much money you need in order to achieve your goals. If that's more than you can earn, break down your goals into smaller, achievable milestones along the way.

How many hours a week? When you're recovering from a serious bout of illness, it can make sense to go back to your old job on a part-time basis—if possible. Alternatively, look for less stressful part-time work to ease back into the workforce.

On the other hand, if you haven't disclosed your illness, initially returning to your old job on a part-time basis could threaten the secret. Only you can judge your capacity and the likely reaction of your employer to a disclosure.

Not too boring, not too challenging or just go for it? As many of us have found, well-meaning people advise us to take an 'easy' job which doesn't challenge us too much. Be careful. A mind-numbing job can send you around the twist in a couple of weeks if you let it. Start out modestly, but go for as much stimulation, challenge and fun in a job as you want. Your self-confidence *will* come back!

GETTING A FOOT IN THE DOOR

Employment placement agencies

These can be a good idea if you're not having lengthy periods of good health, although the waiting list can be years long. You can access local services through social security, public mental health clinics or disability support agencies.

Discrimination during hiring

State equal opportunity laws and the Commonwealth *Disability Discrimination Act* (DDA) make it unlawful for people to be treated less favourably on account of disability. 'Disability' includes 'any condition which affects a person's thought processes, understanding of reality, emotions or judgment or which results in disturbed behaviour'.[4] This includes conditions that are present, have occurred in the past, or might happen in the future. It also covers 'imputed' disability, where people make an assumption that, for example, because we behave in a certain way we must therefore be suffering from a certain condition.

If you think you have been (or are about to be) unlawfully discriminated against, you should contact the Human Rights and Equal Opportunity Commission or your State's equal opportunity or anti-discrimination organisation. Contact details are listed in Appendix III.

To disclose or not to disclose? And if so, when?

It's one thing to share the fact that you have manic depression with someone you trust, but telling an employer is fraught with danger, because employers can have hidden prejudices that can stop you getting a job.

American author David Schneider canvasses some of the options under US law. Quoting Jeffrey G. Allen[5], he says, 'If you have an invisible disability that will not affect any essential functions of your job and will not require an immediate accommodation you need not—and probably should not—say anything.' Not disclosing 'gives you an opportunity to prove yourself on the job. You can feel more confident about disclosing your disability once you have earned the support and recognition of your supervisor and co-workers. The disadvantage of waiting until this time is that you may not be able to do the job well until the necessary accommodations have been made.'[6]

In the same article, Schneider quotes Carol Means, of the US Job Accommodation Network, who sums up the situation: 'It is not necessary to disclose, unless you need an accommodation due to performance problems.'[7]

These principles apply in Australian law, which is similar to the US *Americans with Disabilities Act 1990*, although the terms differ a little. Two key concepts in the Australian law (the *Disability Discrimination Act 1990* or 'DDA') are the 'inherent requirements' of the job and 'reasonable adjustments' that an employer must make to accommodate an employee who has a disability.

Inherent requirements and disclosure In applying for and accepting a job there is only one legal requirement to disclose that we have manic depression:

If we, or our doctors, believe our illness currently prevents us from performing the 'inherent requirements' of the job.

Many people worry about being 'found out' later, and feel that perhaps they should disclose their condition up front anyway. The good news is that the law doesn't require us to disclose, even if our condition is recurring. The Human Rights and

Equal Opportunity Commission states in its information for employers:

> If an employee can no longer perform the 'inherent requirements' of the job because of a disability, you [that is, the employer] will need to look at making workplace changes or adjustments.[8]

Medical examination According to the DDA, employers may lawfully require an applicant to undergo a medical examination. But the medical assessment is limited to determining that the applicant can carry out the inherent requirements of the job, not the applicant's general state of health.

If the medical examination reveals a disability unrelated to the inherent requirements of the job, the employer isn't allowed to refuse to employ you on the basis of the disability. If they do, you can make a complaint to the Human Rights and Equal Opportunity Commission.

Superannuation It's preferable to disclose an illness when applying for superannuation, because the contract usually contains severe penalties for non-disclosure. The super scheme is not permitted to convey the details of your condition to your employer. For more about superannuation see Chapter 11.

Workers compensation You may be asked to sign a declaration stating any prior injuries or illnesses when you commence with an employer. Check the fine print as failure to disclose may mean you forfeit your rights to workers' compensation if work contributes to an exacerbation of your condition.

HOW TO STAY INSIDE

> You come home from work where they've been looking at you sideways for weeks now. The worst thing is the conversation stopping dead when you walk into the room.[9]
>
> Jan Stumbles

Getting sick at work is the stuff of one's worst nightmare. Some of us do it quietly, others spectacularly. What we all have in common is a fear for the security of our job, particularly if our episode caused the boss to learn what was 'wrong' with us.

Ask for 'reasonable adjustments'

If you've had to disclose your condition and you think a 'reasonable adjustment' might help, there's probably not much to lose by seeing if your employer will oblige. In theory, the adjustments can be as varied and as individually tailored as you can imagine. The only thing that can excuse an employer for not making a reasonable adjustment is if it would create 'unjustifiable hardship' for the company.

There have been very few hearings of complaints about psychiatric disability in employment.[10] The reasons for this aren't clear, but a likely factor is people's reluctance to disclose their condition to their employer for fear of victimisation or further discrimination.[11] The result of this is that there are few examples of 'reasonable adjustments' for people with psychiatric disabilities. The following list of ideas might be 'reasonable adjustments' in certain circumstances:

- rostering us on shifts that don't aggravate sleeping difficulties;
- allowing us time off to keep appointments for treatment or support;
- providing workplace accommodation with sufficient daylight;
- varying our hours of work (for example, to accommodate late rising because of sedative medicine);
- adjusting our work or allowing task-swapping so that we're not required to do stressful work;
- providing or funding career counselling or training so we can move to another position or employer;
- providing leave without pay to cover extended periods of illness;

- keeping in contact with us while we're away from work to jointly plan the earliest possible return to appropriate work.

Protect your work reputation

Mary is perhaps the staunchest non-discloser I've met. Mary was struggling to stay at work while battling with the side-effects of a mood stabiliser. She felt faint, nauseated, she had pins and needles and a strange visual sensation. Workmates, who insisted on driving her home, wanted to know what was wrong. 'The flu,' Mary said. And that was that. She was back at work in a day or two, still with side-effects, determined to keep the lid on Pandora's box.

The best bit of advice I've ever received in relation to employment where you haven't already disclosed your condition is:

> *If in doubt about your ability to get through*
> *a day without falling apart, take a day or two off.*
> *Protect your reputation from people's attitudes.*

This is counter-intuitive at first. Surely it would be better to demonstrate commitment to one's work and struggle on? Perhaps, if you have a bad head cold and you can soldier on with a proprietary medicine. But mental illness is different. Every time I go to work when my behaviour and my judgment is 'off', I'm at risk of making mistakes with interpersonal communication, looking ill and generally scaring those around me. Prevailing attitudes to mental illness being what they are, it's often smarter to stay home and 'hide'. The extra time without the stresses of work can also help you recover, rather than deteriorate. Let your own health be more important than other values like commitment or being indispensable.

Use your allies

Ellen and I had practically nothing in common except a mistrust of our boss. But she, surprisingly, with minimal knowledge of mental illness, became one of my staunchest supports when my mental state was deteriorating over a six-month period. Ellen was the one who called a friend to come from another department to sit with me and help me decide to make an appointment with the psychiatrist. Later, she rang me in hospital to pre-warn me that they were considering abolishing my job. We may not all find an Ellen, but even a lesser trusted friend at work can make the difference between losing a job and having enough information to be able to fight for it.

Observe limitations for the public interest

Sometimes the safety of others or the public interest means safeguards have to be put in place. If you can, it's preferable to go along with any regulations or restrictions so you can keep working. For example, Jack is a general practitioner who has manic depression. One of the other doctors in the practice provides professional supervision to make sure that Jack doesn't work if he becomes too ill. Jack's patients can be seen by the other doctors while he's off sick.

Depending on your circumstances, you might have to switch jobs. Mary had a job driving petrol tankers for an oil company. Her employer managed to protect public safety while at the same time not discriminate against her because of her disability.

My doctor knew I was driving petrol tankers and he said that was okay as long as I didn't drive if he thought I was high. I got sick... I was pretty bad, so my husband rang up my boss and told him ...

My boss said it was because of my good record that I was offered another job. But if I hadn't had a good record I would have been out on my ear, because I lied on my medical [questionnaire]... They asked 'Have you got any mental disorders?' and 'Do you take any medication?' The company wanted to sack me because I'd lied on that. I said that it wasn't fair—anyone would do the same in the same circumstances. And they offered me another job.

Some limitations on people with manic depression arise from prejudice alone. As Neil Cole, who was 'outed' and forced to resign as a shadow cabinet minister, said:

> Just because you have a mental illness doesn't mean you are unable to fulfill important roles and functions within society ...There are so many fail-safe mechanisms within our [democratic] armory that we can ensure that any decisions made that may be perceived to be manic or depressive are covered by other mechanisms.[12]

Other limitations are imposed by government regulations, which may or may not be fair. Aviation guidelines used to state that pilots who take lithium were not fit to fly, until the inherent irrationality of this was pointed out (people who *don't* take lithium would be perhaps a higher risk)![13] There are also restrictions on driver licences for people with manic depression—you might be asked by the licensing authority to get a medical assessment as to your driving capacity.

If you're up against an unfair legal restriction, there's little you can do to change things overnight. Try a complaint to the Human Rights and Equal Opportunity Commission, or join a law reform group and lobby for change.

Unfair dismissal

You may be able to take action under unfair dismissal laws if you think you've been sacked for unfair reasons. For example if you're sacked because the employer has discovered your mood disorder, or because your work performance has fallen because you've been unwell, it would be worth seeing if the unfair dismissal laws apply. Contact the Australian Industrial Relations Commission, your union or lawyer as soon as possible.

11

MANAGING MONEY

…he sat down…at the writing-table, to work through the mass of papers, and the contents of a couple of drawers… From her seat at the stove, Louise watched him sorting and reckoning, and she was as grateful to him as it was possible for her to be, in her present mood…Maurice asked her how she had ever succeeded in keeping order, she told him that, before her illness, there had, now and again, come a day of strength and purpose, on which she had had the 'courage' to face these distasteful trifles and to end them. But she did not believe such a day would ever come again.

Henry Handel Richardson, *Maurice Guest*[1]

IMPACTS OF MANIC DEPRESSION ON MONEY

There is a self-evident truth about money and madness: any major mood shift has the potential to cause harm to the wallet. However, between episodes, we resume work, we resume saving, we pay our debts. This healthy period is also a time to take a pragmatic look at the future: is it possible to avoid getting into the same monetary strife again?

It's not that people with manic depression don't know how to manage money. Even those of us who aren't financial wizards know how to budget, plan and save. Money problems arise when our thinking goes 'off'.

Manic spending

There are many spectacular stories about spending during mania and hypomania arising from recklessness or generosity. In the early stages of mania, spending impulsively can feel simply like having fun, capturing something of the playfulness of youth.

Other times we may have an exalted feeling of nobility that comes with generosity and philanthropy. In these stages there are many opportunities to notice the choices we make and, if we're determined, we can decide to lean on the brakes.

Depression and money

According to popular folklore, closed-in depressed people aren't supposed to go on spending sprees, but maudlin generosity and darkly symbolic gift giving is also not unknown among those of us with black mania. Convinced that we won't survive, it seems pointless to keep money in the bank, as Rachel observed. 'I just wanted all the money in my account gone because I didn't plan on coming out of hospital. I didn't think I'd live through it.'

Spending lavishly in this situation is an extreme version of 'retail therapy', one of businessman Rene Rivkin's habits: 'I love money. I love to spend it. I am a great consumer—and when I get depressed, I go out and consume more to try and get me out of it.'[2]

Chaos

Of the many temperamental traits some of us seem to have in common, one of the most infuriating is the tendency to seek chaotic or difficult situations, as if we are addicted to a certain amount of turbulence in our lives. Chaos can work directly on money—the more chaos, the more we spend. If I put off shopping, I know I'll end up at the milkbar for cigarettes instead of planning a trip to the discount smoke shop.

Chaos-making also performs the function of distracting us from being able to think straight enough to pay bills—'I'll pay

A sample budget

	Yearly	Quarterly	Monthly	Fortnightly
Absolute must-pay				
Rent/Mortgage			760	351
Car loan			220	102
Entertainment				50
Mostly unavoidable				
Health Insurance			120	55
Car Insurance	300			12
Contents insurance	250			10
Car registration	450			17
Car running & maintenance	500			19
Car service club	50			2
Ambulance	35			1
Water rates	700			27
Body Corporate fees	400			15
Council rates	500			19
Electricity		180		28
Gas		50		12
Telephone		120		18
Supermarket				150
Petrol				50
Tobacco				80
Alcohol				20
Fares				20
Medical				120
Dental		100		15
Pharmacy			30	14
Childcare				60
Clothing				30
Pocket money				20
School expenses	250			10
Lessons		150		23
Newspapers				15
Books & music			30	14
Hairdresser			30	14
I wish ...				
Savings				50
Holidays	1000			38
Gifts	600			23
			Total	**1,504**

Figure 11.1 A sample budget

that tomorrow when I'm not feeling so disorganised.' The problem is 'tomorrow' gets pushed back day after day until the chaos subsides or a reminder notice—or worse—arrives. Eventually you might arrive at a futile conclusion: 'If events are impossible to foresee, I can't possibly be expected to be able to plan around them, let alone stick to a budget.' However, not keeping track of your finances is an insidious way of shedding your responsibility to look after yourself.

An expensive lifestyle

Like it or not, having manic depression means forking out for expenses that others can avoid. If you're off work and trying to survive for months on sickness benefits, you can find yourself being evicted and having to sell the car to buy groceries.

If you're still working, the cost of medicine and psychotherapy can be crippling. And what about childcare? Many of us leave our children in care outside our work hours so we have a chance to recuperate from the day before collecting them. And that costs money!

Mania brings impulsive buying, generosity and injudicious investing, but we can also run up more subtle expenses. Too many lengthy distance calls and local calls add a layer of misery to the phone bill. The cost of alcohol varies for many of us, increasing with either or both depression and mania.

STRATEGIES FOR CONTROLLING YOUR MONEY

Budgeting

Budgeting's an art, not a science, as I found out (the hard way). Fraught with dangers such as erratic income, not enough income and unexpected expenses, it's enough to give anyone Collingwood supporters' depression.

Here are my ideas of the bare minimum for responsible personal budgeting.

- You have to know how much money you've got—at least twice a week. Luckily telephone banking makes this fairly easy.
- You have to know how much money you owe *now*. Keep all the bills in a single file or folder.
- You have to know how much money you're going to need for future expenses, a year at a time. Keep last year's bills so you can estimate the cost of the coming year's bills.

The rest is simple arithmetic, no magic. Some people use a computer spreadsheet but I prefer to be able to see my budget readily. I use a whiteboard marker and write it on the fridge.

For once-a-year bills, work out what the fortnightly equivalent is and put that money aside. Include car maintenance of $10 per fortnight for a young (less than five years) car and more for an older one.

Arrange your list so you have all the yearly, quarterly and monthly expenses listed together as shown in Figure 11.1. Work out the equivalent fortnightly amounts as follows:

- Turn yearly expenses into their fortnightly equivalents by dividing by 26.
- Turn quarterly expenses into their fortnightly equivalents by multiplying by 4 and dividing by 26.
- Turn monthly expenses into their fortnightly equivalents by multiplying by 12 and dividing by 26.

Add up all the fortnightly amounts. The total is the amount of income per fortnight that you'll need to meet the expenses you've listed. In most fortnights, you will need to put aside these fortnightly amounts for bills that will be due in the future.

Consider how best to put this money aside. You can use a bank account, but this makes it more difficult to keep track of how much money you have accumulated for each of the expenses. If you have a low income, the interest earned on the amount you save can be less than the Federal and State taxes and bank charges that are taken out, and you may find yourself going backwards. As a simple alternative, my mother uses little cardboard tubes which have sturdy lids. She labels each tube 'gas', 'electricity', 'phone' etc., and puts the correct amount of cash in each tube once a fortnight, leaving the money to accumulate until the bill needs to be paid.

Budgeting and saving advice Some financial organisations offer advice on budgeting. However, bear in mind that customer service officers are trained to spot an opportunity to 'cross-sell', that is to sell you another product. You might come away with a special account for saving (including account-keeping fees) when all you wanted was advice.

Watch out for community financial advisors, too. I consulted one when I had been without paid work for several weeks and my ordinary household bills were getting out of control. His advice was that I had only one option: to borrow $1,000 on credit card so as to be able to pay the bills and still have enough for food and accommodation. I resisted that advice, knowing that I would have trouble paying back the credit card debt. I rang all the creditors and arranged to spread out the bills over a period of about five months, leaving me debt-free and with just enough money to survive.

Keeping track of it all Anita has managed her money through illness and health, including managing a successful and highly public business. Her technique, though simple, has been developed over many years. She has a cheap little spirax notebook in which she pencils all her expenditure. She has structured her affairs these days so that she pays for almost every expense by cheque, so she has a record. Her credit union deducts fortnightly easy-plan payments for gas, electricity, water and telephone, and she has arranged to pay for groceries by cheque.

Anita writes up the cheques and, every couple of days, uses the telephone banking service at the credit union to check her balance and to identify which cheques have been cleared out of her account. She told me, 'It only takes about ten minutes every other day or so.'

Debt and creditors

When we're in debt, probably the only way to keep everyone happy is by paying a small part of the amount owing to all creditors over a longer period of time. This way, we can avoid borrowing from a bank or friends. If the debt is huge and catastrophic, you might have to consider bankruptcy (see below).

Creditors are not always polite when you ring to arrange to pay them by instalments, but most are smart enough to know that this may be the only way they'll get their money! Try to overcome the natural tendency to put your head in the sand. Ring them—all they can do is snarl a bit. Alternatively, get a trusted friend or worker to ring on your behalf.

Many companies, including utilities and some private companies, will offer to arrange fortnightly instalment payments. The Australian Tax Office plays fair and is willing to negotiate late payment of a tax debt, although they will impose a penalty.

Bankruptcy This is one of many options increasingly being used by people who find themselves in debt which is impossible to repay.

If an individual has been declared bankrupt:

- creditors are prevented from chasing payment;
- his or her property (except household furniture, certain vehicles and other items) is divided up among creditors;
- restrictions, for example, on borrowing money or being a director of a company, are placed on the bankrupt for a certain period (usually three years); and
- his or her affairs can be investigated.[3]

According to *The Law Handbook*[4], 'The advantages and disadvantages of bankruptcy vary ... and the effects of bankruptcy should be compared with the possible consequences of the debtor not entering into bankruptcy.' If you are considering bankruptcy, seek expert advice from a trusted lawyer or accountant or contact a consumer financial organisation for information (see Appendix III).

Appointing others to manage your money

Enduring Power of Attorney (EPA) This or its equivalent is one of the handiest legal tools, simple and cheap to arrange. An EPA lets you give someone power of attorney over your financial and legal affairs so they can represent you, pay your bills, and even hire someone to continue running your business or start legal action on your behalf if necessary. The beauty of the *enduring* power of attorney is that it stays operational even if you become ill and lose your legal 'capacity' to make sound decisions.

Make an EPA while you're well, choosing very carefully the trusted friend to whom you are giving the power. You can give the power to be operational immediately or, more commonly, to have the power operational only while you are ill or incapacitated.

To be valid, you must understand all the effects of the EPA, including:

- your income and assets;
- that the EPA gives the attorney complete power over your financial and legal affairs;
- that while you're legally competent (of sound mind), you can tell the attorney what to do and how to do it, and you can cancel the power at any time;
- that when you become legally incompetent, the power takes effect and you can't cancel it until you're well again; and
- the attorney's actions won't be audited by any outside body.[5]

You can give a power of attorney to a family member or friend, but consider the possibility that this person might find it an onerous responsibility—or worse, that they might become caught in a conflict of interest. You can get around this by giving your enduring power of attorney to a financial advisor, solicitor or trust company—but be prepared to pay.

If your attorney isn't using his or her power in your best interests, you can apply to the courts for the power of attorney to be cancelled.

Administration order An alternative to an EPA is an administration order, where a court or tribunal orders that someone else is to manage your financial affairs. The relevant court is primarily there to see that we don't get ripped off if we can't manage our money. It can make orders for administration if we have a disability which prevents us from making reasonable decisions and we have a problem that we can't solve unless someone acts on our behalf.

Anyone can apply for an administration order to be made if they believe you've become incompetent to manage your own affairs. The court can make an order that a friend or family member take on the job of administering your affairs. If this is inappropriate, they will make the order to a trustee company. Most orders to trustee companies are made in favour of the State public trustee.

An administration order can be a tyranny or a relief, depending on the efficiency, trustworthiness and understanding of the person who gets the responsibility for managing your affairs. Sometimes it can be disastrous to have a family member (especially one with conflicting interests to your own) to manage your affairs.

Because administration orders are usually made against our wishes, most people hate them and criticise the holder of the order. This is not without some justification—public trustees don't have a particularly good reputation for treating their clients respectfully or in the least restrictive manner.

Administration orders can be revoked by the court that made them and are subject to review by government-appointed auditors. It's also worth noting that the courts can also declare an existing EPA invalid and make an administration order to take its place.

One advantage of the administration order over the EPA is that you have the protection of external auditors and the relevant court to act as umpire. On the other hand, if your administration order is being handled by strangers in a trustee company, you may not have as much say in how your money is spent than if a friend or relative holds a power of attorney.

If you think your administrator is not acting in your best interests or is acting incompetently, you can appeal to the relevant court or tribunal in your State. Check the Order itself for the name of the court or tribunal.

Agreements with a partner Many of us who are in mutually trusting, stable relationships can trust a partner to hold (and not use!) our credit card until we jointly agree it can be used for a specific expense. However, if you change your mind, your partner would be legally obliged to give the card back.

Others adopt a more traditional approach, with the partner with manic depression receiving a share of the household income for personal expenses, leaving bill-paying to the other partner. However, this approach can leave us in a less powerful position. As the power balance swings, the relationship takes on a different quality. Tread carefully and try to retain as much responsibility as possible. If you have to relinquish some responsibility, firmly take it back when you recover.

Bank products

Plastic cards In her practical book *Debt Free*, Anne Hartley's advice is simple: 'If you want to stay out of debt, you have to cut up those credit cards…If you can't give it up, freeze it.'[6]

While credit cards potentially cause more damage, debit-only

EFTPOS cards can be also hazardous because of the easy access you have to your money.

Many people with manic depression don't use plastic cards at all, relying on old-fashioned passbook accounts.

Credit, contracts and manic spending Lots of us have a story that starts, 'I spent so much money when I was high...' These stories are as tragic as they are spectacular. Tragic, not just because we spend all our money or someone else's money, but because we too rarely try to assert our right to get out of the sale contract.

Under the common law in Australia, certain rules for contracts are understood. Among these is the requirement that you have legal capacity to enter into a contract in the first place. 'Legal capacity' includes being of sound mind. If you don't have legal capacity to make a contract, you may be able to get out of it—in certain circumstances. It's more likely you'll be able to get out of a contract if you paid by cash or cheque. If you paid by credit card, the situation is different because your contract was actually made with the bank (not the vendor). If you were not legally incapacitated when you made the credit contract with the bank, your credit contract will stand, regardless of how you used the credit card later. Contracts can also be set aside if the lender knew you had a mental illness that put you at a 'special disadvantage' and enforcement of the contract would be unreasonable or unfair.

Of course, the practicality of getting your money back is not as easy as it should be. You can try speaking to the vendor yourself, if possible, or send a trusted friend. Describe what happened and ask for your money back. Find out if the vendor wondered if you were ill at the time.

If this doesn't get results, conduct a strategic retreat. Consider the pros and cons of doing nothing compared with taking further action. A good place to start getting the information you'll need is a community legal centre, or perhaps you have your own lawyer. Even better, if your State has a mental health legal service you may be able to get advice or representation from them. See Appendix III for contact details.

Keeping your savings safe Some medium-term investments such as 90-day accounts offered by banks have a built-in deterrent to early withdrawal—you lose your interest. However, once I learned that that was the only barrier, and that I could, in fact get my hands on my money immediately, that was the beginning of the end of the only decent sum of money I'd ever had. I needed a safer place for my assets.

I solved the problem by using what was left of the money as a deposit on a place to live. Another way to keep cash safely is by using an *ordinary* Power of Attorney. Give a trusted friend power of attorney specifically for the purpose of your cash management. You can specify that the friend must co-sign any withdrawal from your investment account. This way, your friend has to assess your reasons for wanting to withdraw your money. Watch out with this one, though. It's effective as long as your're prepared to go along with your friend's judgment, but could turn very nasty if you disagree.

Most of us consider savings as the process of building up money in the bank, but when we pay off our borrowings, we're also saving. If you can let go the traditional goal of saving for a large bank balance, you can use any extra money to make payments on long-term borrowings. This is a cost-effective alternative, and in most cases, it is practically impossible to get your hands on the money in the heat of the moment.

Loan consolidation If you have two or more loans, credit cards and store accounts, you'll find you're sending regular payments to the four corners of the earth. The interest rates on all these loans will vary. Consolidating a loan means taking out one mammoth loan with a single lender and paying one 'easy' repayment a month. Do your sums and get a trusted accountant or financial advisor to help or provide advice before you jump into consolidating your loans. You could end up paying much more interest on the consolidated loan than on all the other loans combined.

Regular direct payments Some credit unions will, for no charge, make regular payments to phone, gas, electricity and water companies. This is handy, but you have to watch out you don't withdraw so much that there's not enough left to cover these payments. I solved this one by having two accounts—one for all the 'magic' payments and the other for my weekly expenses and housekeeping.

You can also get your credit union to pay your bills for health insurance, general insurance, phone, gas, water, electricity etc. directly as they come in. The disadvantage of this is you have to remember when all these accounts fall due and make pretty good estimates of how much they will be. If you muck it up, your account could overdraw and/or the creditor's computer will generate a late notice.

Other financial products

Superannuation Most super schemes will automatically enrol a new member for basic death cover. Some automatically enrol new members in basic disablement cover. Most schemes also offer members additional disablement cover for which an extra premium has to be paid. This additional cover is usually subject to a medical questionnaire and/or doctor's report and/or examination. And for people with manic depression, the additional cover is usually rejected or cover is offered at higher premiums. This is legally possible because most insurance policies are excluded from the *Disability Discrimination Act*.[7]

Even if the results of the medical examination show you have been completely healthy, well and in the workforce for years, the simple fact of a previous diagnosis may strike you out. Unfair? Many people think so. If this happens, you can make a complaint under the *Disability Discrimination Act* (see Appendix III for details), but don't hold your breath.

Insurance Insurance seems like an optional extra but the impact of having to use public rather than private psychiatric services or losing your house, its contents, or your car, is huge. If we had enough money to survive on, the loss of any of these would be bad enough. But when you're skint, the impact could be worse and the stress could trigger an episode. Most credit unions offer a fortnightly direct debit for all types of insurance.

LIFE INSURANCE Will your superannuation be adequate for your family if you were to die while they're dependent on you? If you have life insurance or death benefits attached to your superannuation scheme, check the fine print and work out how much your family is entitled to on your death.

Now estimate how much money would be required to keep your family if you weren't alive. Make a yearly estimate for each person for their period of dependence on you. For children, carry this up to their 18th, say, or 25th birthday.

How does the amount you estimated compare with the total pay-out figure from your super? If it's not enough, consider shopping around for life insurance or ask a trusted financial advisor to do this for you. Make sure that there is no suicide exclusion in the policy, if that is relevant to you.

Finally, the questions will be: 'Can I afford this cover?' and 'Can I afford not to have this cover?' Good luck!

INCOME PROTECTION INSURANCE Income protection insurance involves paying a premium for regular or lump-sum payments if you become unable to work through illness or injury. However, it is notoriously difficult to get if you've had treatment for a psychiatric illness. If you're offered cover, expect to pay a higher than normal premium.

HEALTH INSURANCE As well as being an effective safety net, health insurance might be part of your long-term planning to get easier, faster access to hospital services. The health insurance industry has been undergoing significant change recently with Federal Government moves to increase membership. You can get information about the current fees, incentives and rebates from private health insurers.

A Will You can do without a will but it's the only way to make sure that your wishes are actually adhered to. The law is full of bubbly intrigue that can create the most unexpected effects on who gets your money if you don't have a valid will.

You can draw up your own will with a do-it-yourself kit from law stationers and newsagents. These describe the law in plain English and include forms to use for the will.[8]

However, these kits only provide for the simplest provisions, and may not suit your needs. If you have a complex situation (such as stepchildren, or if you want to treat some dependants differently from others), get a solicitor or trustee company to draw your will because the Courts can overturn a will that treats dependants unreasonably.

Legal advice is particularly important if you have reason to believe your will might be contested. Let the lawyer know if this is the case.

Some lawyers and trustee companies charge a fee; others waive the fee in exchange for being nominated as the executor of the will (for which they can charge). This has a few advantages. Solicitors' firms and trustee companies don't die before you, so you know that the firm will still be around when needed. Many people appoint their partner or adult child as executor, but this creates a potential for conflict among family members, and if the executor dies before you, your affairs may be dealt with by someone you would not have wanted to appoint.

12

ADULT RELATIONSHIPS

In this chapter we'll consider the things that can go wrong in relationships when one person has manic depression. We'll look at some of the strategies you can use to preserve or rescue good relationships and minimise the harm from toxic relationships.

It's common in books of this kind to identify the partners in a friendship or relationship as the 'carer' and the 'sufferer'. I think that's quite dangerous, as the terms tend to limit our thinking, reducing whole people to a narrow role. To avoid this trap, I've used the terms sparingly and in inverted commas.

IMPACT OF MANIC DEPRESSION ON RELATIONSHIPS

What it's like for the person with manic depression

I went overseas with a mate and went high. I kept the lid on it with tons of antipsychotics but once we got back home he just kept avoiding me. I was his best mate and he didn't even invite me to his wedding. Some mate.

Jeff

I've drifted away from people who obviously can't cope with [my] mental illness. There are people who you wouldn't tell, and you're not going to get very close friends with them.

Mary

I used to have a high level of respect among colleagues, and lots of people I thought were good friends at that place. But when I heard that one of them was spreading a false rumour that I'd tried to hang myself from the curtain rod in my office, I realised I would never have any credibility among those people again.

Jacqui

It's unnerving to live as if you're in a psychologist's laboratory, with your every move monitored, catalogued and tendered to authorities.

Sheree

My wife's been on the phone to my psychiatrist three times this week. It really pisses her off that he doesn't tell her anything so then she takes it out on me. I should be the one who decides to call him.

Dom

The first time I got sick after we were married, he told me it was all in my head... He'd spoken to the doctor and I'd explained to him what it was all about. But he thought I was alright after that because I was taking lithium, I was cured, I was fine, I wouldn't get sick again. So every time I got sick after that we had these screaming arguments. One time he made a really stupid comment: 'If my father can cure himself of cancer, you can cure yourself of this.' I couldn't trust him properly after that.

Mary

I was undiagnosed until well after Kay left. I was drinking to cover the symptoms but neither of us knew what was going on. Then I got this job in the country and we moved but we didn't last long after that.

Daniel

You can't say exactly how you feel. People try to boost you up. Instead of saying 'Okay, you feel like that', they think 'Where can we go from here?' Probably the best time was when I stayed with my brother and sister for twelve months—they just left me alone. I'd come out of hospital and I went back to work. My sister listened to me. That's very rare. People don't listen because they're too busy giving you advice. My sister didn't push me or try to boost me up or do anything. She didn't say, like my mum used to say, 'Oh give us a smile, Cath' when the last thing you wanted to do was smile. Or 'It's a great day, it must be making you feel better.' That shows the lack in Mum's understanding—although she can do it, she doesn't realise that in depression you can't change your behaviour with a word.

Cathy

My family caused problems because of my irritability and being so demanding being part of the illness—they thought that was me. I think Mum and Dad found it very difficult when they were trying to tell me there was something wrong and I couldn't accept that —'There's nothing wrong, I'm just happy,' that's what I used to say.

I think that to be fair to my first husband, he did try and understand things, but I don't think he ever accepted that I had a psychiatric illness, and that made it hard.

My second husband liked me when I was on a high, probably because my sex drive was really high. I was angry with him because when I met him I was ill and I talked about it and he was able to support me during depression, but he wouldn't accept the fact that I was depressed and would tell me 'Get on with your life'. He used to drink too much anyway and he used to get very aggro and defensive so it was very difficult to catch him to talk at a time when he hadn't had a few drinks.

Jennifer

He keeps reminding me how much of a disaster my illness has been to <u>him</u>. What a cheek!

Mandy

What it's like for those around us

People around us have had a monstrous change forced on them, outside their own control, forcing them to adapt. Like us, they may not want to accept our illness. Like us, they may be angry that the illness has changed us. Like us, they may simply want to wind the clock back to the time when the illness was not part of our lives. Some might expect us to take the blame for the deterioration in our friendship or partnership—others take the blame themselves. People around us grieve for the person they think has left them.

In the thick of the situation, those around us face losses mixed with hopes that things will return to normal. The term 'chronic sorrow' has been coined by researchers to describe the extreme difficulty of grieving over the 'loss' of someone who is still alive but living with difficulties such as a psychiatric disability, brain damage or dementia. In the case of manic depression, this 'death' can be experienced over and over again with each episode, the joy of recovery tainted by fear of the grief that a future episode might bring.

Look what it does to our relationship!

When you're in the midst of an episode or recovering after a crisis, you can easily lose sight of yourself as a whole person. As we necessarily monitor our mood, activity and thinking or become involved in talking therapy, we may end up putting our whole personhood aside in order to focus on surviving.

Before long, we conspire unwittingly with important others to take on roles: we become not 'John and Betty' but 'Carer and Sufferer', 'Giver and Taker'. By unspoken convention, the 'sick' one needs help around home and can't take his or her usual responsibilities. Conversely, the 'carer' becomes magically entitled to blame the 'sick' one for all the extra work/worry/expense involved with the illness.

'Sufferers' feel hassled and resent being told what to do. 'Carers' feel trapped—they didn't ask for this burden but they 'have to' play the role. A 'sufferer' might reject the notion of mental illness while the 'carer' accepts it—or vice versa.

STRATEGIES FOR PRESERVING OR RESCUING RELATIONSHIPS

One positive thing that came out of it for me was forcing me to be more honest and open in my marriage. You do some things when you're high that you probably shouldn't do so you need to be open and hopefully you've got an understanding partner who can see past these things.

Frank

Look for the other person's point of view

Episodes of manic depression can stop us from seeing the other person's point of view fairly, which is essential if we are to preserve or rescue the relationship.

I recognise that I need to consider your point of view without reacting with shame to my contribution to our problems.

In the thick of relationship difficulties it's tempting to lay all the responsibility on the shoulders of the other person. However, I've found I usually have something I can change about myself to improve things. The trick is to recognise where I'm contributing to our problems without getting defensive or beating myself up about it.

Don't act on your present view of the other

An episode of manic depression distorts, selectively filters and magnifies our negative interactions with each other.

> *When one of us is ill, the flaws we usually accept in each other become exaggerated to intolerable levels.*

If you can identify this exaggerated sense of the other person's failings early, you have an opportunity to do a reality check to see if they really are the wicked villain they seem. At this point a useful trick is to stop believing your thoughts. Regard them with mild curiosity but don't act on them or speak from their point of view.

> *Just because you think something, it doesn't mean you have to believe it.*

This trick is especially useful if you're aware that your thinking is going 'off'—if you're becoming suspicious, paranoid or grandiose. Put the idea on hold and check it out with a neutral third party before you act on it or get upset. If you think this sounds difficult, you're right! But it's a technique used by many of the people I interviewed and it is an effective way of preventing damage in all interpersonal relationships. You just have to be well enough to be able to think about 'thinking' and then practise, practise, practise!

Assert your responsibility and limit the roles

The demarcation lines around our responsibility for ourselves are the most important single factor in preserving relationships. Try this imaginary monologue of a person with manic depression talking to their partner or parent.

'If I am allowed to take responsibility for my own life (for example decisions about going off medicine), I can learn from the mistakes I make. If I don't take responsibility for myself (or if those around me make it difficult for me), I can't learn how to recover and I will stay sick.

'You are entitled to your life, free of the millstone of my illness, but you can only do that if your responsibility is *to* yourself and not *over* me. Together, we need to draw the line because if we don't, I will stay sick and you will always have me as your millstone. We will both be angry and our relationship might never recover.

'I can't change how you cope with my illness or your attitude to me but if this causes me problems I will protect myself.

'All I can change is me; only I can decide to change—and I'll only change when the prospect of change becomes less frightening or painful than the status quo. So don't be surprised if I reject your well-meaning advice or resent your well-intentioned intrusion.

'I am grateful that you are prepared to look after me in a crisis and at that time I'll lend you my self-responsibility, but I expect you to give it back when I am well again.'

Reconcile differing views on suicide

When we are at the extreme of despair, contemplation of suicide is logical and internally consistent to us. Our family sees it very differently, of course, but we can't understand how they do not grasp the idea that suicide is simply one of the options in life. Our rationale is incomprehensible to anyone who hasn't seriously entertained suicide.

While it may not be possible for all involved to have the same view of suicide, there is scope for partners in a relationship to learn to live with each other's perspective. Just as divergent political views within a family can be integrated into the family's discourse, differing views on the 'values' of suicide can be resolved.

Let's have a look at some different perspectives on suicide. First, from the point of view of the person experiencing manic depression. Suicide is often sought as the only way to end intolerable pain. When depressed, we believe we are worthless, a burden to others and that the world would be a better place without us. We have no hope of the pain ending; even if we do, we know it can return. Suicide, from this perspective, is not only a courageous thing to do, but is also a noble, self-sacrificing and responsible act.

Second, from the point of view of the person with manic depression who has survived a suicide attempt. After 'waking up alive', we experience mixed emotions. Guilt is common, so is relief at being alive. We might be angry with our rescuers, seeing them as forcing us to stay alive in order that we continue suffering. We have to cope with a barrage of emotions and attitudes from family.

Some families stay away, unable to cope with their own feelings or shamed by the stigma of suicide. Others try to extract promises that we'll never do it again in exchange for pledges to make life better at home. But once we've made a serious attempt, suicide can stay in the back of our minds even when we're well, as an emergency ejector seat. Others, on regaining their health, find suicide has become repugnant and no longer an option.

Third, from the point of view of people close to the suicide. In contrast to the person who is contemplating suicide, the family's view of the world does contain hope. Families do value us, even in the face of our illness. They acknowledge our suffering but see our lives as more than this. They don't want us to leave them. And they want us to think like they do. When we can't adopt their hope or see value in ourselves, our loved ones become frightened and frustrated. They insist. They make deals. Or they give up. Or look for scapegoats. These are all understandable responses from the family's point of view.

Fourth, from the point of view of the community at large. The stigma surrounding suicide influences all of us. Some people try to stage 'accidents' to spare their families the additional grief and pain they know would be caused by obvious suicide. Bereaved families strain under the taboo, some only referring to the suicide as 'death'.

The significant thing about these four very different perspectives is that they are each valid. Partners in a relationship can reconcile differing attitudes to suicide if they both recognise the validity of the other person's point of view. The fact that each party has a different point of view does not mean that either of us is wrong; nor should anyone's view be required to change. Both the survivor and the family may need to put in a great deal of difficult personal emotional work if their relationship is to emerge without permanent damage.

RELATIONSHIPS THAT WERE DETRIMENTAL IN THE FIRST PLACE

Families have been unjustly blamed for causing mental illness, and this must stop. But the fact that things which happen in families can strongly affect mental health cannot be ignored.[1]

The only thing I could do was to put a huge distance between them and me, so I moved interstate.

Paul

My son has a right to see his grandparents. But at what a price to me! I didn't have contact with my mother until he was three—I knew I wouldn't cope if I saw her again, and sure enough I ended up in hospital. I rang her about a month ago but only after I'd discussed it in therapy for weeks.

Jasmine

My brother suicided a few years ago, so when I get badly depressed, the pressure's really on from Mum.

Rory

This guy I lived with was bashing my kids and playing mind games with me. Getting intervention orders didn't make a scrap of difference. Then he wrote this dreadful letter to my seven-year-old. And made a totally fictitious, malicious complaint about my mum that nearly destroyed her career. You just can't keep living with people like that if you want to survive.

Mandy

Some of us know clearly who our enemies are and how they operate to destabilise us. Others, including those who have been abused or traumatised, may not at first see clearly that the stress is coming from a toxic relationship.

With some thought and watchfulness, we can start to connect mood shifts and crises that appeared to come 'out of the blue' with real events in our lives. For some, these events could be contact with a certain family member; for others, it might be an event that unsettles us disproportionately more than expected. If we look closer, we may find that the recent event has the hallmarks of an earlier experience, perhaps forgotten until now.

Of the damage that comes from other people, the most significant appears to come from those who have known us longest and who have had positions of power over us—our families of origin. Ironically, it is often to our families of origin that we look for our closest support and affirmation and it is this that can trap us in a Catch-22 situation.

Mental health workers often deny that families can be damaging, especially if they are in contact with those family members! If you're lucky enough to have a psychiatrist or mental health worker who places you (not your 'carer') in the centre of the picture, they may be able to help you protect yourself from interactions that damage you.

Beating blame

One of the most upsetting impacts of manic depression on relationships is the audacity with which people seem to blame us for our condition. On one hand, people insist that we are 'ill'. The process of illness is fortuitous, by inference not caused by human misdeed. This allows people to feel pity for us as sufferers of misfortune, and removes any source of guilty feelings they might accord themselves if they believe they may have had a hand in our misfortune.

Yet, in an amazing flouting of logic, the same people punish us with disrespect, leaving us to conclude that as opposed to believing we are 'ill', they actually subscribe to ancient ideas that we must have done something bad so the gods are punishing us.

The best strategy I've found for beating blaming messages is to remember the 'shoulds'. Don't insist to yourself that other people *shouldn't* blame you for being ill or your behaviour when ill. Let them. They'll be the ones who get upset.

13

MUMS, DADS AND KIDS ON THE ROLLER-COASTER

No parent can guarantee a child a trouble-free journey through life, although we might wish to try. In this chapter I want to consider what we know of the children's needs and share some ideas that people with manic depression use when bringing up their children.

HOW MANIC DEPRESSION AFFECTS OUR KIDS

The opportunities

When we're well, people with manic depression are normal parents. Manic depression can also be an advantage to us as parents. Having to learn how to cope with traumatic events and battle on forces us to lead more considered lives. We develop a perspective on life that acknowledges the inevitability of human suffering and we teach our children from that understanding.

Along the way, we learn that even major setbacks aren't usually fatal and we can readily use that knowledge to teach our children to pick themselves up after small catastrophies. We apply in parenting the psychology we've learned in the course of our own journeys; our lives focus on continuing development.

The challenges

Like it or not, when manic depression is active it affects those around us, including our children. Though most studies of the effects of manic depression on kids tend to focus on the negatives and use questionable frameworks and methodology,[1] it's worth considering some of the 'risk factors' that have been identified.

Our fluctuating ups and downs and periods of normal good health mean it's hard to provide a consistent emotional environment for children. A depressed view of the world can lead us to be pessimistic about our own future and our children's endeavours.

Studies also conclude that some parents with major depression put a guilt trip on their kids, saying things like, 'If you'd stayed home from school today to look after me, I wouldn't have had to go to hospital.'

The research indicates that we also tend to be over-protective. We may be prevented by illness, separation and sedation from 'switching on and tuning in' to our kids, leading many researchers to conclude that we have trouble bonding with our kids and letting them separate to become individuals.[2]

None of us likes the grains of truth contained in these studies, but don't get defensive! Consider whether the negative effects are happening in your family. If they're not happening, that's terrific. If they are, the knowledge gives you power to change things.

From my knowledge of parents with manic depression, I think that most of us manage to minimise the damage our condition can cause. What follows is an adaptation of mainstream common sense and conventional parenting wisdom applied to the needs of our children.

STRATEGIES FOR PARENTING WITH MANIC DEPRESSION

What do the kids need?

Table 13.1 lists some of the key elements that our kids may need. The list isn't exhaustive and has been compiled from private research as well as recent studies.[3]

What the children need
To understand their parent's condition
For their parent to acknowledge their fears
To have skills to cope with their life as it is
To be free from shame, blame and other toxic talk
To have someone who has already earned their trust
To know there are other families like theirs
To have the very best of their parent who has manic depression
To have a life of their own, take risks and have lots of fun!
Minimum disruption when their parent is ill
To be free from looking after their parent

Table 13.1 Needs of children who have a parent with manic depression

To understand their parent's condition Kids have a need to know, in terms they can understand, what's going on. For a preschooler, draw an analogy with the changing weather, or with the child's own experiences of anger, sadness and happiness. I invented a couple of terms: 'pokers' were little sudden bothers, like pricking your finger with a needle; and 'waves' were big strong surf waves that push you over and you get scared in the water. It's okay that they know you get scared from time to time. You can show them by example how to cope with fear.

Remind the children that in time you'll be *yourself* again. Remind yourself by repeating it to them.

For their parent to acknowledge their fears As the children grow you can introduce more detail, more explanation and comments about how you feel about the episodes. Their capacity to formulate questions and identify their own feelings grows with them, so be increasingly prepared to listen and acknowledge their experiences of the crises.

To have skills to cope with their life as it is Go out of your way to encourage assertiveness in the children. Encourage them to tell you about their fear—whether it's a fear of your rage or that you're no longer the parent they know, love and yearn for.

Teach them what you've learned—relaxation, visualisation, assertiveness, cognitive techniques, your philosophical position as long as it's not toxic.

To be free from blame, shame and other toxic talk Tell your child, over and over that he or she couldn't possibly have caused your manic depression, even if it started when they were born.

Whatever you do, don't say things that are toxic. You know the sort of stuff, you've heard it yourself. No guilt trips. No blame. Gracious suffering. Withdraw if you have to. When they ask 'why', don't blame anyone, including God or yourself. Say 'I don't know' if you don't know. Keep the toxic stuff for a journal. If you express shame about your illness, you teach the children to be ashamed too. Find something, anything will do, that you can be proud of that counteracts your sense of shame. It might be, 'I'm pretty good at bouncing back after these episodes', or 'I usually get my understudy in quickly to limit the child's fear', or 'I'm following all the paths to good health that I know of', or even 'I can show my child a model of suffering that will help him or her in later life'. Show them you don't care (even if you do care mightily) if people snub you because you're ill. Tell the kids you're sad that Mrs X doesn't seem to understand and perhaps she's afraid, too.

If something shaming, blaming or plain toxic slips out (and it will, we're only humans and we're suffering superhuman pain), correct yourself as soon as you can. Encourage them to say what they felt when you uttered the toxic words, and acknowledge it.

To have someone who has already earned their trust I reckon this is the critical bit that is overlooked by authorities. An adult stranger who appears in a crisis saying to a kid, 'Trust me to look after you—your Mum or Dad obviously can't', isn't going to win the kid's confidence without a lot of hard work.

Make sure that doesn't happen by helping the youngsters form ongoing relationships with grandparents, neighbours, teachers, aunts and uncles, and your friends. Then, in a crisis, the children already know they have other trustworthy adults around to rely on.

One way of formalising this is to arrange for a willing person who has already earned your children's and your own trust to become your understudy when you're ill. Someone who can, if necessary, move in to your home and take over where you have had to leave off. This way, your understudy can be the means by which the children can keep their usual routines and their own lives ticking over; the understudy can do everything you do around the house; and the children will be less likely to come to the attention of child protection people.

Another important step is to (without self-blame) *expect* that the children will have difficulty coping with the problems created by your crises. Get them counselling before any behavioural problems arise. Counselling can help them cope, and also give you ideas on how to help them. Many parents worry, realistically, that if we seek counselling for our children we are admitting we can't be good enough parents.[4] Certainly, the prevailing view among social workers and clinicians attached to mental health services is that any psychiatric illness in us automatically means our children are at risk, even though this has been debunked by Burdekin[5] and other respected researchers.

To be on the safe side, get counselling help for the children through channels that are independent of mental health or child protection services. In any case, enlightened workers will see that by taking the initiative for our kids, we are actually demonstrating mature, effective parenting.

To know there are other families like theirs Whether your child goes to a formal program for children of parents with mental illness or just gets to meet your adult friends who also happen to live on the roller-coaster, it's important for them to know that other kids have troubles too. Don't force the issue—it's often enough for them simply to meet another kid who has a parent with a similar problem.

To have the very best of their parent who has manic depression Share yourself with the children. Share the things you find fun; participate in the things they like to do. Have fun with your kids—you are allowed to, you know! Do with them your favourite activities—sewing, cooking, sport, travel, going shopping, to the bush, the beach, the movies, playing with the dog or a kite in the park. Give them a go at stuff, no strings attached. Try new things together, enjoy rainy-day rituals, whatever they are in your family.

Help them 'unpack' emotionally after a crisis and do something for fun. There's no need (and it can be damaging) to shower them with gifts ('bribes') after a crisis—this can reward their looking after you, or give them the idea that you are ashamed of your illness after all.

Nurture their self-esteem: encourage rather than praise them; give consequences rather than punishment; listen and acknowledge; give them boundaries. (See Further Reading.)

To have a life of their own, take risks and have lots of fun Let the children be themselves. Remember that genes and temperament play an important role in determining how kids 'turn out'—it's not just down to the parents' behaviour. Let them separate, remind them that they have choices all the way.

The child's life is as important as yours. Not more, nor less. They will become themselves with or without our blessing and encouragement. Give them boundaries but let them take risks. Protect them from toxins while you show them what you've learned from your experiences.

Teach them St Francis' prayer (see Chapter 8) or make up your own together: 'Dear God, I'm pissed off that Mum gets sick and it's not fair. I can't do much about Mum getting sick but could you give me a cuddle when I need it and let me have fun like all the other kids?'

Let them go and they'll come back. Be proud of your work as a parent but know that your child is, ultimately, himself.

When the kids are living with you

Minimum disruption when their parent is ill Prepare safety nets and plan in advance so that when you reach a critical point, your child can be looked after. Try to arrange it so the kids are with someone they already know and trust and, just as importantly, keep them at home, in their own routines, with their pets, friends, school and beds. Use your understudy as a key person in your safety net team.

To be free from looking after their parent Watch carefully and call on your understudy. Adults who've grown up with mentally ill parents are unanimous on the long-term damage caused by having had to look after Mum or Dad.[6]

We had a mantra in our family: 'It's Mum's (or Dad's) job to look after you and it's your job to have fun.' As they grow, the mantra can change to acknowledge the children's increasing capacity and responsibility for housework, pets and school work: 'It's everyone's job to look after their own responsibilities (and have fun)—but Mum's (or Dad's) health is not your responsibility.'

Parenting from a distance

Improving your chances of having the children return There are some things you can do to improve your chances of having the children return to live with you. The most important are:

1. Recover your health.
2. Rebuild your life.
3. Re-establish your credibility in the eyes of the people who have the power to determine with whom the children live.

Learn what the 'experts' say about parenting; do a parenting course; join a support group of other parents whose children don't live with them. Do lots of stuff with your kids (even though it might take you a week to recover after a short visit!).

Keep the house clean and tidy when the children and/or social workers visit—get some help with housework if you need it. Make sure the fridge contains milk, fruit, veggies and meat. Get rid of your stash of empty beer bottles. Be sober. Be as alert as the medicine allows. Appearances *do* count.

Coping with children's absence Elsewhere I've written about the devastation brought about by the discriminatory attitudes and processes by which society removes our children from us,[7] here I want to focus on how we can deal with separation from our children.

Paul's wife won custody of their young son on the basis of Paul's mental illness. He told me:

I went into hospital and that was the last I saw of my son. She just upped stumps. I tried to find them for years. Sometimes I have to stop looking for him because it gets too painful and aggravates my illness. So I stop and concentrate on me, my health. I'll have another go next year. But I'll find him—eventually.

Don't waste your energy being cross. Focus on getting well. Turn the separation into rest, recreation and healing time. Focus not on getting them back but on rebuilding your life. A year or so after my interview with Paul, his son, now a teenager, contacted him, wanting to get to know the Dad he'd lost. During the separation, Paul had concentrated on rebuilding his life. He's been back on track for some time, with good health, steady employment and accommodation, and he's in a strong position to be a Dad again.

Don't desert young children—they didn't abandon you. Keep up whatever contact you are allowed, and push for more contact when you can.

Grieve that you can't be around to support your children, even if you fear for their safety:

> I had to agree to my daughter living with her father. There wasn't any other option. I worry how she'll cope living with her father because my marriage was very emotionally abusive.
>
> Veronica

If you have contact by phone or letter, you can offer them a supportive lifeline even if you can't directly alleviate their woes. Support them if they are having problems with their other parent or foster parent, and teach them ways of coping, but don't criticise the other person to the child. Take action through adults if your child is at risk.

Mourn the lost opportunities to teach them your values directly and find creative ways of giving them your love and support. You *can* show them your unconditional love from a distance; you can demonstrate to them your values by how you conduct your life and your contact with them and their current carers. You can demonstrate patience and persistence in the face of difficulty; you can show them by example how to deal with setbacks of their own.

Be patient All kids evaluate their parents at some stage, whether or not the parents have been ill. As our kids approach adulthood and as they mature as adults or as parents themselves, their opinions of us change as their insights into our own situation develop. In a television interview in 1998, broadcaster Jessica Rowe reflected on her childhood with her mother, Penelope Rowe. She said, 'It didn't matter that she [was depressed and] couldn't [cook or do the housework]—because she's such a great mum.'

Above all, remember that children grow to make their own choices. They may choose to blame us (they wouldn't be alone, but that wouldn't necessarily make them right!). They may choose to forgive us. The choices are theirs to make, not ours to demand.

TO BREED OR NOT?

If you're diagnosed with manic depression after your children have been born, the question of whether to have children is irrelevant, but people who are diagnosed before having children can be confronted with conflicting advice. You might choose not to have children because of the many 'what if?' questions that arise. If the 'what ifs?' are bothering you, it might help to remember the dangers of 'awfulising' and the trap of telling yourself you couldn't survive if such-and-such an event occurred (see Chapter 5). Here's a list of 'what ifs' that people consider.

What if the children get manic depression?

Many, including Kay Redfield Jamison, a world expert clinician on manic depression and also a 'sufferer', would answer, 'What if there was no manic depression in the world?' As genetic research progresses, scientists may soon be able to identify foetuses that are at high risk for developing manic depression. Jamison is concerned that this could lead to expectant mothers with manic depression being advised to terminate their pregnancies. She points out the danger of tossing the baby out with the bath water[8]—we might rid the world of mania and depression and in doing so lose the variety of characteristics that have given us fine and inspirational leaders and artists.

In any case, the chance of your child developing Bipolar Mood Disorder is only about one in seven[9] and leading experts don't recommend avoiding having children on this score.[10]

What if I get ill during the pregancy?

Plan the pregnancy not only with your partner but also with your mental health worker or psychiatrist. Discuss the pros and cons of using medicines during the pregnancy. Organise extra safety nets.

If you become pregnant unexpectedly while you're taking medicines, get medical advice immediately you suspect you might be pregnant, but don't despair. Medicines that pose the most danger to the baby probably won't affect it. For example, lithium causes birth defects in 5–10 per cent of babies, which means there's a 90–95 per cent chance of the baby *not* being affected.

What if my relationship breaks up?

Sure, life will get tough for a while, but it won't kill you.

What if they take the children away or my non-manic-depressive partner gets sole custody?

Have a look at the ideas about living away from your kids. Get legal advice about your rights.

What if I can't counteract the negative effects of my condition on the children?

No parent can guarantee their child a trouble-free passage through life. The best you can do is the best you can do—so do that, and enjoy your children.

14
MYSTIC OR MANIC?

It is inevitable that trauma of any kind can raise questions about religion or spirituality, and manic depression is no exception. What is exceptional, though, is the systematic denial of the relevance of these questions to people with 'mental illness'. In this chapter we look at how manic depression can impact on spirituality and faith and how some people draw on faith to assist their recovery. We also consider how to cope with the community's denial of spirituality and the conundrum posed by religious or spiritual experiences that coincide with episodes of manic depression. I should state at the outset that I make these remarks from the basis of my own spiritual tradition—protestant Christianity.

IMPACTS OF MANIC DEPRESSION ON FAITH AND SPIRITUALITY

The devil...can upset and disturb the soul...by bringing impure thoughts into the person's mind. If the soul takes any notice of these they can cause it great harm... The devil manages to make them see very vividly, in their minds, dreadful and impure things. Sometimes these things are even closely linked to the spiritual things and people which have been beneficial to their souls...You should feel particularly sorry for people who have a melancholic disposition, since they suffer from these attacks most severely.

St. John of the Cross[1]

Can manic depression make faith wither?

Many of us find illness can challenge our faith or our sense of God.

I lost my concept of God for a long, long time—He went out the window when I became unwell...and it's only really come back in a very fragile sense...I'd like to believe more, but I don't. So I go to Mass, and I enjoy the Scripture and I enjoy the music and in communion there is a certain amount of meaning to me but it's just at a very rudimentary stage. And maybe my faith won't develop any further.

Veronica

Wendy's faith survived her illness, but as she pointed out:

It's hard enough working out what God wants me to do anyway, without psychosis complicating things.

Can manic depression cause faith to grow?

Angela hints at a link between faith in oneself and faith in a higher being:

Mental illness certainly has an impact on faith and spirituality. I feel I have a greater faith due to Bipolar because I have overcome major obstacles and continue to do so.

Frank has had two manic episodes, in both of which he believed he was Jesus Christ. Frank's manic experiences as Jesus seem not to have hampered his later growth in faith:

I found it increased my spiritual awareness—even though I had mania that was related to being an important religious figure. Before that I wasn't atheist but I didn't really have any faith. Once I got sick, not so much at first, but after a period of time, I developed some faith in God (whatever God is for whoever, that doesn't matter). I believe that there is a higher source now, but before that, I didn't know.

After Frank had told us about his growth of faith, I asked him how it had happened.

Because I became Jesus Christ! (laughter) Actually I think it's because you've been punched in so low, or maybe before I was too proud to recognise. I was brought up in the Christian Brothers College, attended Mass, a strong Catholic origin. I probably didn't take it all in—I was too 'smart' for all that. And because I got so low (even though I don't go to Mass every Sunday or go to confessions now), I've got a great faith now that I never had in my life.

Frank is pointing to the 'leveling' or humbling experience of manic depression as a factor in his experience of growth in faith.

Some thoughts on 'sin'

Most of us have experienced other people's belief that our moods, activities and thoughts when unwell are sinful, bad, slothful or manipulative! But do we need to agree with them and beat ourselves up because of it? Do we need to confess, ask forgiveness or feel guilty?

One of the most enlightened ideas the church gave to me was that sin was, fundamentally, a state of separation from God. In this sense, depression *is* sinful—the experience of disconnectedness with all persons, including God. If this is the case, we can acknowledge the fact of our state simply, without blaming ourselves for something that is beyond our control.

There is little that is purely 'wrongdoing' in depression, although that is not to say that as we mature and recover we often become aware of being able to change some things about ourselves.

IMPACTS OF SPIRITUAL EXPERIENCE ON MANIC DEPRESSION

If our condition can impact on our spirituality, we can equally find that faith, beliefs or spiritual practices can impact on our condition.

How spiritual experience can be helpful

Martin, who had a problem with violence when he was in a hypomanic or mixed state, found that meditative prayer every day helped his overall level of stress, and this, combined with talking therapy and medicine, reduced the danger of his mood shifts. I've found that I can manage mood shifts a little easier if I can get to a creek or a park for twenty minutes, to reconnect with the natural world.

Among the people I have spoken to, spiritual practices are important for our overall well-being, although few rely on faith or religious beliefs alone to manage their manic depression. Spirituality's healing effects can be seen in preventing us from coming to harm.

As Paul told me:

I met a guy in the street who I'd never met before in my whole life and he said to me, 'Did you hear God?' He didn't even introduce himself. I said 'What do you mean?' He said that when he slashed up he heard God booming in his head and he had to get to the nearest house to get help.

This story bears a striking resemblance to Jonathan's:

I was at work [in the lab] and it got so bad that I decided that I would mix up a glass of cyanide and kill myself. I got the cyanide down, and I got a beaker, and of course it's forbidden to use laboratory stuff to drink from, so I was very careful to wash a glass (to make sure I wouldn't poison myself before I put the cyanide in it). I got halfway through washing the glass when I heard God say to me, 'Go and ring your parents and have tea there tonight.' The way God speaks to me is a cross between just a voice and a feeling, but it's recognisably different from an internal thought—it definitely seems to be coming from outside... So I went up to my parents and collapsed into tears at the table. They took me to hospital that night.

Suffering

Suffering has heightened my everyday appreciation for life.

Angela

I sometimes compare suffering with weight training. Mighty weightlifters were all once tiny babies who could barely manage to lift a toy block to their mouths. As they grow, and add a training regime, their muscles strengthen so they can lift heavier and heavier objects. At the peak of a weightlifter's career he might be able to lift more than 200 kilograms.

It's the same with suffering. We have small pains that are at first difficult to bear. We may have also large pains that we are not strong enough to fend off. Yet each time we use our 'pain-lifting' muscles, we are strengthened for the next time. After going through pain, such as manic depression, or divorce, or loss of a child, we often find that when little issues come up, we can lift them as easily as the baby learns to lift his block.

Always look on the bright side, and other bunkum William James,[2] writing at the turn of the twentieth century, considered that people fell into two groups: the 'Healthy-minded' and 'Twice Born'. 'Healthy-minded' people like to live on the surface of life, and don't understand suffering, its purpose or those who suffer. Their goal is happiness and they don't even seem to notice negative stuff, except to say 'tut, tut ain't it awful'. In some individuals, says James, 'the capacity for even a transient sadness ... seems cut off from them as by a kind of congenital anaesthesia.'[3]

James criticises the church of his day for 'a victory of

healthymindedness.'[4] 'Repentance, according to ... healthy-minded Christians means *getting away from* the sin.'[5]

These ideas are echoed by later writers:

> There is a popular image of piety which seems deliberately to exclude most, if not all, of the negatively toned emotions. The Christian is seen as one who ought to be full of love, joy, peace, patience, kindness, goodness, faithfulness, gentleness and self-control (Galations 5:22). We are not like this, of course, but we feel we ought to be, that there is something wrong with us or lacking in our faith if we allow the negative emotions to intrude into our lives.[6]

The Monty Python team expresses 'healthy-mindedness' best in *The Life of Brian*, in which the thieves being crucified with Brian/Christ sing along, 'Always look on the bright side of life'.

Much of the ordinary worship in churches across Australia is also well-described by 'healthy-mindedness', but as each of us knows, this attitude is an inadequate anchor in a life of turbulence.[7] The fact that 'bad stuff' is present in our lives means we are forced to recognise it—we cannot escape it, and we must make sense of it.

William James' other group of people, the 'Twice Born', is aware of evil and darkness around them. Most of his examples are of people who suffered melancholy, including Tolstoy, Bunyan and Luther. 'In the religion of the twice-born', says James, 'peace cannot be reached by the simple addition of pluses and elimination of minuses from life.'[8]

What does this mean for us? Firstly, I think it can help explain people's behaviour in response to our illness. All the friendships I've lost or tossed out since I had problems with mood disorder, and all the people who have distanced themselves from me have one thing in common: their 'healthy-minded' attitude to life. On the other hand, people I am drawn to these days and those who have stuck with me are 'twice born'.

Secondly, being made aware by depression or mania of the darker side of the world gives our spiritual side a rich experience to work with and, unlike our 'healthy-minded' friends, to make sense of the operation of evil around us.

Rites of passage Whether our suffering arises from the desolation of depression, thoughts of suicide or the social consequences of our illness, we plumb depths not known by others and, because of this, we're forced to explore what despair means, if anything. Can a period of despair enhance our relationship with God? For some Christians, a period of spiritual dryness is necessary for our ongoing journey towards God, according to the medieval monk, St. John of the Cross, who coined the phrase 'dark night of the soul'.

> ... some of these people [with melancholia] are able to prevent the devil's attacks when they try really hard [but] they do not usually shake themselves free of this until their own mental disposition is cured, unless the dark night enters the soul and so expels all of its impurities, one by one.
>
> St. John of the Cross[9]

St. John of the Cross specifically excluded depression resulting from the external world from this 'dark night'. But does major depression, as an experience that isn't a reaction to external events, fit the description? Can the soul enter this 'dark night' through the vehicle of major depression? Can major depression be a true spiritual dryness through which we may take steps toward God? I can only wonder at possible answers to these questions, and hope that there is interest among mystic Christians to teach us more openly about these things.

Harmful religious messages

Of course, there are instances in which religious messages or our beliefs can aggravate our condition or prevent a full recovery:

A lot of people are ill because of the false religious beliefs that they've picked up. So psychiatrists have to get rid of these false beliefs that people hold ... this doormat Christian stuff.

Jonathan

I was in the Navy hospital for about four weeks ... they told me I was self-destructive and probably had endogenous depression and the medical officer in charge told me that the only way I was going to be saved would be if I turned to God. I told him he was talking garbage.

Mary

Some religious messages can be harmful for someone experiencing severe depression. When depressed, we have lost our usual resilience and a call to 'Confess and Repent!' can see us believing literally that we are hopeless sinners now that we lack our previous capacity for hope. Also, when deeply depressed, we know we cannot *do* anything to change our state of mind, so that when called on to repent, or turn to Christ, we are immobilised. Yet the insistence of the minister continues unabated, providing more 'evidence' to our depressed eyes that we have indeed no worth in either God's, others' or our own eyes. We conclude we are no good and can be no good.

When we're unwell, our 'sin' is not misdemeanour but separation from God, and it is often not within our mental or spiritual power to reduce that separation. Accordingly, messages of 'Turn to Christ' should be replaced by messages of 'Await His Grace'.

Coping with religious messages Remember that even benign messages can take on damaging effects if we receive them while our thinking is 'off'. If you have a trusted friend who you can talk to about religion or spirituality, you can ask that person to help you to follow the 'discernment' guidelines (see below).

Keep alert for damaging messages and brain-washing techniques, whether they are unintentional or deliberate, regardless of whether they come from the pulpit, self-help groups or the family.

PSYCHIATRY AND SPIRITUALITY

> Faith, I believe, has a very minute place in psychiatry. I've never heard it mentioned in my thirteen years' involvement with psychiatrists.
>
> Angela

Even though psychiatry's diagnostic linchpin, the *Diagnostic and Statistical Manual of Mental Disorders*[10] (DSM-IV) recognises the occurrence of religious themes in mania, discussion of religious or spiritual matters between mental health workers, psychiatrists and their patients is minimal. The amount of discussion in psychiatric literature about the apparent overlaps between madness and the spirit world is negligible. Freud viewed religion as 'a system of wishful illusions together with a disavowal of reality, such as we find ...nowhere else...but in a state of blissful hallucinatory confusion'.[11]

Albert Ellis, founder of Rational Emotive Therapy, is even more radical:

> All humans...have some kind of philosophy...but some religions claim that we derive ethics from God or from some supernatural entity. But religiosity ... means a devout belief in the supernatural ... one God ... that tells us exactly what you should do, and if you do that you will have a good life and if you don't you will be damned.[12]

Ellis here is speaking out against 'the god who said "should"'. (Actually, God does nothing of the sort: to the contrary, he created Eden and let people choose their own way.) At least Ellis recognises that religious messages that say 'you should' ('thou shalt') can be damaging to people.

Carl Jung wrote:

> I never try to convert a patient to anything, and never exercise compulsion. What matters most to me is that the patient should reach his own view of things. Under my treatment a pagan becomes a pagan and a Christian a Christian, a Jew a Jew, according to what his destiny prescribed for him.[13]

Jung's work is rarely practiced these days in mainstream ('biological') psychiatry, although a few psychiatrists, psychologists and clergy draw on some of his principles. In Australian mental health services, the standard professional line is 'individuals who bring religious and spiritual problems into their treatment are often viewed as showing signs of mental illness'.[14] The lack of a diagnostic category that distinguishes mystical from psychotic experiences leads to the treatment of all 'symptoms' (regardless of their psychotic or mystical natures) with psychotropic medicine. Paul wisely kept this mystical experience from his mental health workers:

> I hadn't been well, and I'd lost just about everything … I remember being down at the beach, depressed, and I was abusing the hell out of whoever rolled the dice and decided what path my life would take. I was so angry. And then there was an overwhelming not-knowing what to do next. There was just nothing else that I could try. And it was like feeling 'Why was this life given to me? What's this? What's the very core essence of why I exist?'
>
> And then I remember looking at the city and that to me represented the whole world and it felt like I was expected to take on the whole world. You gotta be kidding. There's no way I'd be successful at that.
>
> And then there was this sort of knowing. It wasn't like someone speaking, no voices or anything like that, it was just a knowing that what was expected was to try, not succeed or fail, just try. And that's all that mattered and if I did that,

that's all that mattered, and that would give my life purpose. If I didn't try, that was the most rejecting of the things that I'd been given.

The attitude of psychiatry as a profession to spiritual matters is unsurprising when we learn that, according to one study, psychiatrists as a group are far less religious than the general population.[15] I would suggest that this applies also to the population of psychiatric nurses and other mental health workers.

You can cope with anti-spiritual attitudes in the treatment of manic depression by choosing carefully to whom you talk about spiritual questions. Find like-minded people from among those with manic depression; look to your church congregation; read and pray.

MYSTIC OR MANIC?

In the middle of an episode we can be presented with all sorts of spiritual difficulties. Some of us hear voices during psychotic mania (up to 47 per cent of episodes, according to one author[16]) and even those who don't hear voices can be torn between accepting the experience as mystical or categorising the experience as pathological. An early study suggested that religious themes occur in 29 per cent of manic episodes.[17]

How do we interpret these experiences? Are they spiritually authentic? Or are they totally fictional and without basis? Are they just symptoms? Although psychiatry is generally indifferent to this question, a few researchers have given it some thought, among them David Lukoff.[18] Despite R. D. Laing's observation that although 'experience may be judged as invalidly mad or as validly mystical... the distinction is not easy',[19] Lukoff came up with the idea of separating mystical experiences while allowing an area of overlap.[20] In the overlapping area are 'Mystical Experience with Psychotic Features' and 'Psychotic Disorders with

Mystical Features'. Examples include Carole's experience of being drawn to the church whilst suffering a manic episode, Frank's manic experience of becoming Jesus Christ and Jonathan's experience in the lab. Paul's experience on the beach was simply a mystical experience.

Mystical experiences with psychotic features are characterised by the presence of certain themes: death, rebirth, journey, spirits, cosmic conflict, magical powers, new society and divine union.[21] Lukoff suggests that a 'positive outcome' is likely if the following features are present: wellness before the episode, sudden onset of episode, triggered by stress and the person viewing the episode as 'meaningful, revelatory, growthful.[22] On the other hand, a psychotic episode with mystical features would have a less positive outcome.

Although Lukoff was writing some years ago,[23] the DSM-IV[24] has not incorporated his ideas. Further, as he points out, 'neither psychologists nor psychiatrists are given adequate training to prepare them to deal with [psychospiritual] issues.'[25]

The church, too, often has difficulty interpreting our experiences. Matthew Fox points out that 'the denial of mysticism by churches and synagogues is a deep and enduring scandal'.[26] Graeme Griffin put it this way: 'Most of the major denominations in our time seem to have as much difficulty in coping with ecstasy as they do with agony.'[27] Ironically, the views of modern psychiatry that uphold 'mental illness' and deny 'spiritual experience' are often echoed in the pulpit and the confessional.

Many church leaders at the parish level have not been educated in issues to do with mental illness, let alone considered the co-existence of experiences of both illness and mysticism. Although some churches have a long tradition in doing things for the mentally ill, such as running hospitals, the services they provide are based on a secular psychiatry that denies spiritual wisdom.

Coping with the overlap—'Discernment'

Both church and psychiatry have 'forgotten' how to discern helpful from dangerous mystical experiences, but works from medieval times do have something to say about this dilemma. St. Teresa of Avila and her pupil St. John of the Cross taught the skill of 'discernment' or distinguishing. That this is important is underlined in the first letter of John:

> It is not every spirit, my dear people, that you can trust; test them, to see if they come from God.
>
> 1 John 4:1[28]

There are several means by which we can protect ourselves from the effects of spirits whether or not they are masquerading as symptoms of mental illness.

Do not actively seek mystical experiences In *The Ascent of Mount Carmel*, St. John of the Cross advises that 'the soul should resist revelations ... there is no need to desire to receive goods in a way that is supernatural and beyond one's capacity.'[29]

Discuss your experience St. John of the Cross tells us to get to 'an experienced confessor or to a discreet and wise person'[30] who can help us identify dangerous experiences. This is particularly important if you think you could be in the 'Dark Night of the Soul'—it could equally be that you are dangerously depressed.

Only act on the experience if it's benign and authentic Authentic, benign spiritual experiences:

- enhance the gifts of the holy spirit;
- promote humility;
- do not impair your ability to reason;
- keep you generally within your own spiritual tradition; and
- don't preoccupy you.[31]

HOW TO INTEGRATE SPIRITUAL TRUTHS INTO LIFE ON THE ROLLER-COASTER

If psychiatry is unwilling to take our spirituality seriously and the mainstream church is unable to grasp mysticism or psychosis, we will have to teach them. In small, organic groups we can propagate these ideas and pray that they will be taken up. We can also use established mechanisms to call on religion and psychiatry to work with us to find ways in which they can acknowledge our experiences and thereby guide us in improving and maintaining our spiritual and mental health.

In the meantime, we need to protect ourselves with silence, carefully seeking others who share or who are sympathetic with our experiences.

CONCLUSION

So you're at the end of the book and you might still be wondering, 'Yeah, this is easy for you to say, Madeleine, but I still can't see that things can improve. It's not that I haven't tried, but I'm not getting anywhere.'

Don't try this stuff if you're overwhelmed by trauma. Look after only the coldest penguins and wait. Stay alive. The very fact that you picked up this book means you're on your way. Even if you seem to forget everything you've read, even if you think it's codswallop, something useful might be germinating in your mind. Every conversation, every book, every waking up to a variation in well-being, every choice, every problem addressed, every disaster that falls adds up to a rich experience that you can draw on *when you're ready.*

If you are seeing some improvement in your quality of life, I only have one final caution, expressed best by Emily Dickinson:

> *Is bliss, then, such abyss,*
> *I must not put my foot amiss*
> *For fear I spoil my shoe?*
>
> *Poems Third Series* 1896

In other words, don't let your vigilance spoil your fun.

Learn again how to relax, play and be spontaneous; take a

risk and have a rest from constant self-vigilance; dare to experience joy without bubbling over into a high.

Follow your interests and your capacity. Whatever allows you to follow your dreams can be the source of a well-rounded, unlimited life. Ask yourself, 'How much fun can I get away with?' rather than 'I wonder if I'm up to that?' By now, you'll have worked out many strategies to limit the potential of manic depression to ruin your fun—now's the time to put them into good use!

If you can see some light at the end of the tunnel, don't worry about oncoming trains[1]—it's probably daylight. Follow it and feel the warmth!

APPENDIX I—JARGON DECODER

A glossary of medical, psychiatric and nursing words and phrases[1]

Acute 'Sudden' or 'short-lived'. Not to be confused with 'severe'. See also *Chronic.*

Affect Term used by psychiatrists. Refers to mood and emotion—swinging, flat, blunted, appropriateness, and type for example, anxious, elevated, depressed, suspicious, irritable, guilty etc.

Anorexia Lack of appetite.

Antipsychotic Type of medicine used to eliminate symptoms of psychosis.

Anticonvulsant Type of medicine used to eliminate seizure activity, also used to stabilise mood.

Benzodiazepines Class of medicines used for their anti-anxiety, anti-mania and muscle relaxant properties. Known to be addictive if used over an extended period.

Biorhythm Natural body rhythms such as the sleep/wake cycle, and the menstrual cycle.

Bipolar Literally 'two poles,' refers to mania and depression as two extreme states.

Borderline Personality Disorder Disorder of the Self, developmental in origin, often associated with early trauma. May be more common in sufferers of manic-depressive illness.

Case manager Nurse, occupational therapist, psychologist or social worker employed by mental health service to provide primary care to people with mental illness as a 'one-stop shop'.

Cerebral Of the brain.

Chromosomes Tiny structures, made up of genes, inside all body cells.

Chronic Occurring over a period of time. Not to be confused with 'severe'. See also *Acute*.

Circadian rhythm Daily rhythm or cycle.

Clinically depressed Depressed, the judgment having been made on the basis of taking a history and examining the mental state of a patient.

Co-dependency Unwittingly getting your jollies from someone else's problem while they do the same to you.

Cognitive To do with thinking.

Cognitive behavioural therapy Talking therapy that modifies behaviour (and mood) by acting on the patient's thinking.

Compliance Used by psychiatry to denote whether we are taking prescribed medicine.

Contraindication A condition which makes it dangerous to prescribe a given medicine, for example, 'Lithium is contraindicated in pregnancy.'

Delusion A thought not based in reality, a false belief.

Denial Protective defence mechanism.

Depression Painful and potentially dangerous state characterised by lowered mood, sluggish thinking and lowered levels of activity.

Diagnosis Determination of the nature of a disorder.

Discharge plan Plan made before discharge by patient and clinical staff about recovery after leaving hospital.

Disinhibited More reckless than usual.

Dysphoria Malaise, unpleasant state of mind. Opposite of euphoria.

Dysthymia Low-grade chronic depressed feelings.

Elation Normal human emotion; also a sign of mania. Elation alone is not mania.

Electroconvulsive therapy (ECT) Practice of sending electrical impulses through the brain. Used in the treatment of depression and also for acute mania.

Episode Period of acute unwellness.

Euphoria Pleasant state of mind. 'Eu' prefix means good, well, normal, but 'Euphoria' is also used to denote abnormally elevated mood.

Familial Runs in families, but not necessarily genetically inherited. See also 'Genetic'.

Genetic Inherited characteristic. In the case of manic depression, an inherited vulnerability.

Hallucinations A sensory experience that doesn't belong to ordinary reality. More common during episodes of mania, hallucinations also occur during severe depression. A 'psychotic' phenomenon (along with delusions).

High Plain English term for mania or hypomania.

High dependency Usually locked section of psychiatric hospital where people are held who are out of control, violent, at risk of suicide or self-harm or a risk to others, or who are vulnerable to other patients.

Hypersomnia Sleeping too much. Can occur in the depressive phase of Bipolar illness.

Hypomania Literally 'little mania'. Pronounced hypO-mania ('hyp*er*-mania' isn't a word).

Hyposomnia Not sleeping enough.

Inhibitors Chemicals, including medicines, that inhibit or stop the action of other chemicals in the body.

Insight-directed therapy Talking therapy that aims to heal by helping the patient understand and get insight into their situation.

Insomnia Disturbed sleep pattern; also meaning 'not sleeping at all'.

Irritability Mood state that can accompany mania, hypomania and depression.

Labile Fluctuating or unstable.

Low Diminutive term for 'depression'.

Major Depression Psychiatric term for depression that meets DSM-IV diagnostic criteria.

Mania Potentially dangerous state where hyperactivity, invincibility, a vision or mission, persuasiveness and risk-taking behaviour can lead to disaster or death.

Manic depression Collection of conditions characterised by episodic mood shifts and associated changes in activity and thinking. Includes Bipolar I, Bipolar II, Major Depression, Cyclothymia and Dysphoric Disorders.

Melancholia Traditional term for depression and manic depression.

Mental illness Specific term applying to psychoses (for example, manic depression, schizophrenia) and neuroses (for example, obsessive-compulsive, panic and other anxiety disorders, eating disorders etc.). Excludes personality disorders and brain disorders. See also 'Psychiatric Condition'.

Monoamine oxidase inhibitors (MAOIs) Class of antidepressant medicines that work by inhibiting the action of the enzyme called 'monoamine oxidase'.

Mood Aspect of human experience that is altered in manic depression. Psychiatrists categorise mood as being stable or 'labile' (see above), appropriate or inappropriate, blunted, flat, or restricted in scope. 'Mood' includes being elevated, depressed, suspicious, irritable, guilt-ridden, anxious, perplexed.[2]

Mood swing Term of unknown origin suggesting that having manic depression is as much fun as being on a swing in a playground. Try saying 'mood shift'.

Motor retardation Slowed-down physical movement associated with severe depression.

Neuroleptic Class of antipsychotic medicines.

Neuron A cell of the brain and nervous system that communicates with other neurons by firing electrical charges by the chemicals they produce. Medicines used by psychiatry act on neurons and their chemical 'transmitters'.

Neurotic A sub-type of mental illness, covering non-psychotic illnesses such as anxiety disorders. A neurosis is a condition connected with reality and is like an overreaction to events around oneself. Also derogatory term meaning 'whinger'. See also *Psychotic*.

Neurotransmitters Chemicals produced by neurons (see above) to send messages around the brain and nervous system. Many medicines act on neurotransmitters.

Nystagmus Involuntary flickering of the eyes. Can be caused by some psychiatric medicines.

Occupational therapy Discipline that believes the activities we do can assist healing.

Over-inclusive thinking Having better than usual ability to see connections between things. In the eyes of psychiatry, this is a symptom.

Paranoia False ideas, usually suspicious, jealous or blaming in nature about being treated specially or singled out for harassment or, less commonly, as a hero.

Personality Set of typical behaviour and thinking patterns unique to an individual.

Personality disorder Label used to describe a person's condition when their typical patterns of behaviour and thinking (that is personality) are maladaptive.

Phobia Irrational fear.

Post-natal After birth.

Post-partum After having given birth.

Prophylactic Preventive.

Psychiatric condition Catch-all term for conditions treated by psychiatry and includes mental illnesses, personality disorders and brain disorders. See also 'Mental Illness'.

Psychiatry Leading academic and professional discipline in the developed world that defines, researches and treats 'mental illness' and 'psychiatric conditions'.

Psychology Scientific and professional discipline concerning itself with the function of the human mind.

Psychosomatic Symptoms experienced in the body but which arise from the mind.

Psychotic A psychosis is the loss of touch with reality. It might mean having hallucinations and/or delusions. A subtype of mental illness, psychosis occurs in illnesses such as schizophrenia, manic-depressive illness, schizo-affective disorder and others. Pyschosis in manic depression may occur during a manic episode ('manic pyschosis') or during depression ('pyschotic depression').

Puerperal Refers to the period immediately after giving birth.

Rapid cycling According to DSM-IV, rapid cycling is four or more episodes in a year. See also *Ultra-rapid Cycling*.

Rational Emotive Therapy (RET) Type of cognitive behavioural therapy (see above) developed by Albert Ellis. See Chapter 5.

Refractory Unresponsive to treatment.

Response Improvement following (that is as a result of) treatment.

Restraint Physical approach, such as holding the patient down etc., carried out to restrain a patient.

Schizophrenia Treatable mental illness characterised by disturbances of thought and perception and may include psychotic symptoms of hallucinations and delusions.

Seasonal affective disorder Type of manic-depressive illness that is worsened in winter.

Seclusion The act of putting a patient in a small room without windows which is locked from the outside.

Secondary depression Depression that occurs because of some other event (as opposed to apparently coming 'out of the blue').

Secondary mania Mania that occurs because of some other event (as opposed to apparently coming 'out of the blue). Can occur as an unwanted effect of treatment, for example in HIV/AIDS therapy.

Serotonin reuptake inhibitors Class of antidepressant medicines that inhibit the action of the enzyme that mops up the serotonin produced by neurons.

Side-effects Unwanted actions of prescribed medicines.

Sign A sign is something that *other people* experience as a result of our disorder—an *objective* as opposed to a *subjective* experience. For example a sign of mania is sleeplessness. See also 'Symptom'.

Somatic Bodily.

Somewhere safe May be used as a euphemism for nursing practices including restraint, high dependency and/or seclusion.

Specialling Nursing practice whereby one nurse is assigned to be with a certain patient for the entire shift.

Stupor A state of near-unconsciousness with little thinking or responsiveness going on. Can accompany depressed and mixed states.

Suffer To bear up.

Suicidal State of thinking about, or planning suicide.

Symptom A symptom is something we experience or suffer. For example, we might feel restless during mania—that's a *symptom.* (Others can't experience our restlessness but they may observe that we do not sleep—that's a *sign.* See also *Sign.*)

Synapse Connection between neurons.

Tardive dyskinesia Involuntary, incurable rhythmic 'munching' movements of the face and mouth caused in some people by some antipsychotic medicines.

Temperament Supposedly in-built approach to life, for example happy-go-lucky, intense, fiery.
Toxic Poisonous.
Ultra-rapid cycling Recently 'discovered' fast fluctuations in mood. See also 'Rapid Cycling'.
Unipolar Former term for Major Depression.

APPENDIX II—
MENTAL HEALTH ORGANISATIONS

These organisations' contact details were as published at the time of writing, but if you find the phone numbers are incorrect, phone Telstra Directory Assistance.

CRISIS

National
Lifeline Ph: 13 11 14

REFERRAL

National
SANE Australia Helpline
Ph: 1800 688 382

Mental Health Information for Rural and Remote Australia
Ph: 1300 785 005

Australian Capital Territory
ACT Mental Health Crisis Team
Ph: 02 6205 1065 or 1800 629 354

Victoria
Emergency department of nearest public hospital

Tasmania
Campbell House TAS Referral Number
Ph: 03 6234 2802 9am–5pm
Extended hour paging 016 181 405

South Australia
SA Mental Health Crisis Team
13 14 65

Western Australia
WA Mental Health Crisis Team
Ph: 08 9227 6822

Northern Territory
NT Mental Health Crisis Services
Darwin: Ph: 08 8999 4911
Alice Springs: Ph: 08 8981 9227

Queensland
Salvo Care Line Counselling Service
Brisbane: Ph: 07 3831 9016
Sunshine Coast: Ph: 1300 363 622

ORGANISATIONS OF 'CONSUMERS' FOR 'CONSUMERS'

National
Australian Mental Health Consumers Network
PO Box 222 Coorparoo QLD 4151

Track down other groups via SANE Australia
PO Box 226 South Melbourne VIC 3205
Ph 03 9682 5933
www.sane.org/

Aussie Consumer Newsletter at www.vicnet.au/~aussiecn

Victoria

MoodWorks Educational Society Inc.
PO Box 424 Deepdene DC VIC 3103

Geelong Bi-Polar Support Group Inc.
139 Yarra Street Geelong VIC 3220
Ph: 03 5222 5999

North Eastern Bipolar Support Group
Ph: 03 9464 6455

Mood Disorders Support Group
c/- Mental Health Foundation (Victoria)
270 Church Street Richmond VIC 3121
Ph: 03 9427 0406 Fax: 03 9427 1294

Consumer groups that are members of the Victorian Mental Illness Awareness Council Inc.
c/- 23 Weston Street Brunswick VIC 3056
Ph: 03 9387 8317

South Australia

Consumer-only groups that are associated with the Mood Disorders Association (SA) Inc,
1st floor, Mental Health Resource Centre
1 Richmond Road, Keswick SA 5035
Ph: 08 8221 5166

Queensland

'Consumer-led support groups' and 'Peer advocacy program'
c/- Queensland Association for Mental Health
20 Balfour Street New Farm QLD 4005
Ph: 07 3358 4988

ORGANISATIONS FOR CHILDREN

Australian Association for Children of Parents with a Mental Illness
c/- Prahran Mission, PO Box 81 Prahran VIC 3181
Ph: 03 9510 6750

National Network of Adult and Adolescent Children who have a Mentally Ill Parent/s. Vic. Inc (NNAAMI)
PO Box 213 Glen Iris VIC 3146
Ph: 03 9889 3095

OTHER MENTAL HEALTH ORGANISATIONS

National
SANE Australia
PO Box 226 South Melbourne VIC 3205
Ph 03 9682 5933
www.sane.org/

Mental Health Council of Australia Inc.
PO Box 174 Deakin West ACT 2600
Ph: 02 6289 8039 Fax: 02 6289 7703

Mental Health Foundation (Australia)
266 Church Street Richmond VIC 3121
Ph: 03 9427 0407

Australian Capital Territory
Mental Health Resource
Ph: 02 6287 4214

Victoria
VICSERV, Psychiatric Disability Services of Victoria (peak body)
370 St. George's Road,
Fitzroy North VIC 3068
Ph: 03 9482 7111 Fax: 03 9482 7281

Tasmania
Tasmanian Association for Mental Health
111 New Town Road New Town TAS 7002

South Australia
Mood Disorders Association (SA) Inc,
1st floor, Mental Health Resource Centre
1 Richmond Road, Keswick SA 5035
Ph: 08 8221 5166

Mental Health Resource Centre
1 Richmond Road Keswick SA 5035
Ph: 08 8221 5166

Western Australia
Association for Mental Health
305/79 Stirling Street Perth WA 6000
Ph: 08 9420 7277

Northern Territory
Central Australian Mental Health Association
PO Box 2336 Alice Springs NT 0871
Ph: 08 8981 4128

Queensland
Queensland Association for Mental Health Inc
20 Balfour Street New Farm QLD 4005
Ph: 07 3358 4988

APPENDIX III—
OTHER USEFUL ORGANISATIONS

These organisations' contact details were as published at the time of writing, but if you find the phone numbers are incorrect, phone Telstra Directory Assistance.

MONEY

National

Banking Industry Ombudsman
Ph: 1800 337 444

Australian Consumers Association
Ph: 02 9577 3399

Superannuation Complaints Tribunal
Ph: 13 14 34

New South Wales

Credit Helpline
Ph: 1800 808 488

Australian Capital Territory

CARE Financial Counselling and Consumer Credit Legal Service
Ph 02 6257 1788

Victoria

Credit Helpline
Ph: 03 9602 3800 or 1800 803 800

Consumer Credit Legal Service
Ph: 03 9670 5088

Tasmania

Anglicare
Ph: 03 6334 6060

South Australia

Adelaide Central Mission
Ph: 08 8202 5180

Western Australia

Financial Counsellors' Resource Project (referral)
Ph: 08 9221 9411

Northern Territory

Anglicare Top End
Ph: 08 8985 0000

Queensland

Queensland Financial Counselling Association
Ph: 07 3209 3622

LAW AND COMPLAINTS

National

Human Rights and Equal Opportunity Commission
GPO Box 5218 Sydney NSW 2001
Ph: 02 9284 9600 or 1800 021 199

Federal Privacy Commissioner
GPO Box 5218 Sydney NSW 1042
Ph: 1300 363 992

Commonwealth Ombudsman
Level 5 1 Collins Street Melbourne VIC 3000
Ph: 03 9654 7388 or 1800 133 057

Telecommunications Ombudsman
Ph: 1800 062 058 Fax: 1800 630 614

New South Wales

Disability Discrimination Law

Disability Discrimination Legal Centre
Shop 99, 1–5 Meeks Street Kingsford NSW 2032
Ph: 02 9313 6000

Legal Aid
Legal Aid Commission of New South Wales
PO Box K847 Haymarket NSW 1238
Ph: 1800 806 913

Medical Board
Medical Board of New South Wales
PO Box 104 Gladesville NSW 1675
Ph: 02 9879 6799

Equal Opportunity and Anti-Discrimination Agency
Anti-discrimination Board
181 Lawson Street Redfern NSW 2016
Ph: 02 9318 5444 or 1800 670 812

Health Complaints
Health Care Complaints Commission
Ph: 02 9219 7444

Australian Capital Territory

Disability Discrimination Law

Disability Discrimination Legal Service
Havelock House, Gould Street Turner ACT 2612
Ph: 02 6247 2018

Legal Aid

Legal Aid Commission
4 Mort Street Canberra City ACT 2601
Ph: 02 6243 3411

Medical Board

Medical Board of the Australian Capital Territory
PO Box 1309 Tuggeranong ACT 2901
Ph: 02 6205 1599

Equal Opportunity and Anti-Discrimination Agency

Human Rights Office
GIO House, City Walk Canberra ACT 2601
Ph: 02 6207 0576

Health Complaints

Health Complaints Unit
Ph: 02 6205 2222

Victoria

Mental Health Law

Mental Health Legal Centre Inc.
Level 4, 520 Collins Street Melbourne VIC 3000
Ph: 03 9629 4422 Fax: 03 9614 0488

Disability Discrimination Law

Disability Discrimination Law Advocacy Service Inc.
GPO Box 1139K Melbourne VIC 3001
Ph: 03 9602 4877 or 1800 651 275 Fax: 03 9602 4979

Villamanta Legal Service Inc.
6–8 Villamanta Street Geelong West VIC 3128
Ph: 03 5229 2925 Fax: 03 5229 3354

Legal Aid
Victoria Legal Aid
350 Queen Street Melbourne VIC 3000
Ph: 03 9629 0234 or 1800 677 402

Medical Board
Medical Practitioners Board of Victoria
1 Palmerston Crescent South Melbourne VIC 3205
Ph: 03 9695 9500

Equal Opportunity and Anti-Discrimination Agency
Equal Opportunity Commission of Victoria
380 Lonsdale Street Melbourne VIC 3000
Ph: 03 9281 7111 or 1800 134 142 Fax: 03 9281 7171

Health Complaints
Health Services Commissioner
Ph: 03 8601 4199

Tasmania

Disability Discrimination Law
Launceston Community Legal Centre Inc
4A George Street Launceston TAS 7250
Ph: 03 6334 1949

Legal Aid
Legal Aid Commission of Tasmania
GPO Box 9898 Hobart TAS 7001
Ph: 1300 366 611

Medical Board
Medical Council of Tasmania
PO Box 8 South Hobart TAS 7004
Ph: 03 6223 8466

Equal Opportunity and Anti-Discrimination Agency
Human Rights and Equal Opportunity Commission
4A George Street Hobart TAS 7000
Ph: 03 6234 3599 or 1800 001 222

South Australia

Disability Discrimination Law
Norwood Community Legal Service Inc.
110 The Parade, Norwood SA 5067
Ph: 08 8362 1199

Legal Aid
Legal Services Commission of South Australia
82–98 Wakefield Street Adelaide SA 5000
Ph: 1300 366 424

Medical Board
Medical Board of South Australia
PO Box 359 Stepney SA 5069
Ph: 08 8362 7811

Equal Opportunity and Anti-Discrimination Agency
Equal Opportunity Commission
30 Wakefield Street Adelaide SA 5000
Ph: 08 8226 5660 or 1800 188 163

Western Australia

Mental Health Law
Mental Health Law Centre (Western Australia) Inc
217 Beaufort Street Perth WA 6000
Ph: 08 9328 8266

Disability Discrimination Law
Sussex Street Community Legal Service Inc.
29 Sussex Street East Victoria Park WA 6101
Ph: 08 9470 2676 or 1800 642 791

Legal Aid
Legal Aid Western Australia
GPO Box L916 Perth WA 6001
Ph: 08 9261 6222

Medical Board
Medical Board of Western Australia
PO Box 1040 West Perth WA 6872

Equal Opportunity and Anti-Discrimination Agency
Equal Opportunity Commission
141 St Georges Terrace Perth WA 6000
Ph: 08 9264 1930

Northern Territory

Disability Discrimination Law
Darwin Community Legal Service
17 Peel Street Darwin NT 0800

Legal Aid
Northern Territory Legal Aid Commission
Cavenagh Street Darwin NT 0800
Ph: 1800 019 343

Equal Opportunity and Anti-Discrimination Agency
Human Rights and Equal Opportunity Commission
80 Mitchell Street Darwin NT 0800
Ph: 08 8981 9111 or 1800 810 815

Queensland

Disability Discrimination Law
Welfare Rights Centre Inc.
11th floor, 295 Ann Street Brisbane QLD 4000
Ph: 07 3864 8511

Legal Aid
Legal Aid Queensland
GPO Box 9898 Brisbane QLD 4001
Ph: 1300 651 188

Medical Board
Medical Board of Queensland
GPO Box 2438 Brisbane QLD 4001
Ph: 07 3225 2524

Equal Opportunity and Anti-Discrimination Agency
Anti Discrimination Commission of Queensland
50 Ann Street Brisbane QLD 4000
Ph: 07 3239 3365 or 1800 068 305

Health Complaints
Health Rights Commission
Ph: 07 3234 1674 or 1800 077 308

FURTHER READING

CHAPTER 1

Personal accounts

Cronkite, Kathy *On the edge of darkness* Doubleday New York 1994
Dowling, Bary *Mudeye* Wakefield Press Kent Town South Australia 1995
Duke, Patty *A Brilliant Madness* Bantam Books New York 1992
Jamison, Kay Redfield *An Unquiet Mind* (first published Alfred A Knopf New York 1995) Vintage Books New York 1996
Millett, Kate *The Loony Bin Trip* Simon & Schuster New York 1990
Millett, Kate *Flying* Touchstone (Simon & Schuster) New York 1990 (first published Knopf New York 1974)
Orum, Margo *Fairytales in Reality* Pan Macmillan Australia Sydney 1996
Rzecki, Catherine *Surfing the Blues* HarperCollins Publishers (Australia) Sydney 1996
Styron, William *Darkness Visible—A Memoir of Madness* Random House New York 1990

CHAPTER 2

Bishop, Lara *Postnatal Depression: Families in Turmoil* Halstead Press Sydney 1999
Bloch, Sidney and Singh, Bruce S. *Understanding Troubled Minds: A guide to mental illness and its treatment* Melbourne University Press Melbourne 1997
Grounds, David and Armstrong, June *Ecstasy & Agony—Living with mood swings* (2nd edn) Lothian Melbourne 1995
Mueser, K. and Gingerish, S. *Coping with Schizophrenia* New Harbinger Publications, California 1994

Veggeberg, Scott K. *Medication of the Mind* Allen & Unwin Sydney 1996 (First published Henry Holt & Company, New York 1996.)

CHAPTER 4

Bloch, Sidney and Singh, Bruce S. *Understanding Troubled Minds: A Guide to Mental Illness and its Treatment* Melbourne University Press Melbourne 1997.

Carter, Warwick *The Australian Home Guide to Medicine* Redwood Editions Melbourne 1997

Grounds, David and Armstrong, June *Ecstasy and Agony* Lothian Melbourne (2nd edn) 1995

SANE Guide to Treatments SANE Australia PO Box 226 South Melbourne Victoria 3205

Veggeberg, Scott K. *Medication of the Mind* Allen & Unwin Sydney 1996 (First published Henry Holt & Company New York 1996)

CHAPTER 5

Talking therapies

Bernard, M. E. *Staying Rational in an Irrational World* McCulloch Melbourne 1986

Berne, E. *Games People Play* Grove Press New York 1964

Ellis A. and Harper, R. *A new guide to rational living* Whilshire Books North Hollywood CA 1975

Harris, T.A. *I'm OK—You're OK* Pan London 1973

Complementary and alternative therapies

Damian, Peter and Damian, Kate *Aromatherapy—Scent and Psyche* Healing Arts Press Vermont 1995

Geddes and Grosset *Guide to Natural Healing* David Dale House New Lanark Scotland 1997

Hochhuth, Klaudia *Practical Guide to Reiki: An ancient healing art* Gemcraft Melbourne 1996

Williams, Tom *The Complete Illustrated Guide to Chinese Medicine* Element Books Brisbane 1996

CHAPTER 6

Melbourne Consumer Consultants' Group Inc. *Do you mind? The ultimate exit survey: Survivors of psychiatric services speak out* Melbourne Consumer Consultants' Group Inc. Melbourne 1997

CHAPTER 8

Jamison, Kay Redfield *Touched with Fire—Manic Depressive Illness and the Artistic Temperament* Free Press New York 1993

McKay, Matthew and Fanning, Patrick *Self-Esteem* New Harbinger Publications Oakland CA 1987

CHAPTER 11

Hartley, Anne *Debt free* Doubleday Sydney 1992

James, Vivienne *The Woman's Money Book* Anne O'Donovan Pty Ltd Melbourne 1996

Newell, Malcolm *Ten steps to financial health* Stirling Press Adelaide 1995

CHAPTER 12

For people who care about someone who has manic depression

Berger, Diane and Lisa *We heard the angels of madness: A family guide to coping with manic depression* New York Morrow 1991

Dinner, Sherry *Nothing to be ashamed of: Growing up with mental illness in your family* Lothrop, Lee and Shepard Books New York 1989

Golant, Mitch and Golant, Susan K. *What to do when someone you love is depressed* Henry Holt & Co New York 1996

Johnson, Julie Tallard *Understanding Mental Illness: For teens who care about someone with a mental illness* Lerner Minneapolis 1989

Oster, Gerald D. and Montgomery, Sarah S. *Helping your depressed teenager* Wiley New York 1995

SANE Australia *Carer's Handbook—Caring for someone who has a psychiatric disability* 1996

SANE Australia *The Sane Guide for Brothers and Sisters—A guide for siblings of people living with a mental illness* Melbourne 1998

Secunda, Virginia *When Madness Comes Home* Hyperion New York 1997

Skynner, Robin and Cleese, John *Families and how to survive them* Cedar London 1993 (first published Methuen London 1983)

Woolis, Rebecca *When someone you love has a mental illness* Tarcher/Putnam New York 1992

For everyone

Berne, Eric *Games People Play* Grove Press New York 1964

Bloch, Sidney and Singh, Bruce S. *Understanding Troubled Minds: A guide to mental illness and its treatment* Melbourne University Press Melbourne 1997

Jansen, David, and Newman, Margaret with Carmichael, Claire *Really relating* Century Hutchinson Sydney 1989

Lerner, Harriet Goldhor *The Dance of Anger* Harper & Row New York 1985

West, Morris *Vanishing Point* Harper Paperbacks New York 1996

CHAPTER 13

For parents

'Children and Parents' in Barnard, Michael E. *Staying Rational in an Irrational World* McCullough Publishing Carlton 1986

Kelly, Madeleine 'Approaching the last resort: a parent's view' in Vicki Cowling (ed.) *Children of Parents with Mental Illness* Australian Council for Educational Research, Melbourne 1999

McKay, Judith 'Building Self-Esteem in Children' in *Self-Esteem* Matthew McKay and Patrick Fanning, New Harbinger Publications Oakland CA 1987

Sayce, Liz 'Parenting as a civil right: supporting service users who choose to have children' in A. Weir and A. Douglas *Child Protection and Adult Mental Health—Conflict of Interest?* Butterworth-Heinemann Oxford 1999.

For teenagers

Dinner, Sherry *Nothing to be ashamed of: Growing up with mental illness in your family* Lothrop Lee & Shepard Books New York 1989

For teenagers who are depressed

Cobain, Bev *When nothing matters anymore—A survival guide for depressed teens* Free Spirit Publishing Minneapolis 1998

Garland, E. Jane *Depression is the pits but I'm getting better* Magination Press Washington DC 1997

For children

About manic depression

Kelly, Madeleine 'Wendy Weatherbane and the Rainbow Angels' (unpublished) 1998

About other conditions

Laskin, Pamela and Moskowitz, Addie Alexander *Wish upon a star: A story for children with a parent who is mentally ill* Magination Press New York 1991

Liddicut, Jan *Is Dad Crazy? An explanation of schizophrenia for children* (illustrated by Linda McKay) Schizophrenia Australia Foundation, Melbourne 1989

Sessions, Deborah *My Mom is Different* Sidran Press, Sidran Foundation for Mental Illness Lutherville MD 1994 (about multiple personality disorder)

For mental health professionals

Cowling, Vicki (ed.) *Children of Parents with Mental Illness* Australian Council for Educational Research, Melbourne 1999

Weir, A. and Douglas, A. *Child Protection and Adult Mental Health—Conflict of Interest?* Butterworth-Heinemann Oxford 1999

CHAPTER 14

Estes, Clarissa Pinkola *Women who run with the wolves* Random House Sydney 1993 (first published Rider London 1992)

Fox, Matthew *Original Blessing* Bear & Company Santa Fe New Mexico 1983

Fox, Matthew *The Coming of the Cosmic Christ* HarperCollins New York 1988

Grof, S. and C. Grof (eds) *Spiritual Emergency* Tarcher Putnam New York 1989

Lowenthal, Kate M. *Mental Health and Religion* Chapman & Hall London 1995

Watkins, John *Hearing Voices, A Common Human Experience* Hill of Content Melbourne 1998

REFERENCES

Grateful acknowledgement is made to the following for permission to quote from the following copyrighted material. The publishers and author have made every effort to contact all holders of copyright material included in *Life on a Roller-Coaster.* They would be pleased to hear from anyone who has not been duly acknowledged.

PREFACE

1 Brown L. (ed.) *The New Shorter Oxford Dictionary* Oxford 1993 p1730
2 ibid
3 ibid
4 Dementia praecox was renamed schizophrenia by Emil Bleuler in 1911. Source: Goodwin, F. K. and Jamison, K. R. *Manic-Depressive Illness* Oxford University Press New York 1990 p.101
5 By its third edition, the *Diagnostic and Statistical Manual of Mental Disorders* (American Psychiatric Association, Washington DC 1980) the term 'manic depressive illness' was replaced by other terms.

CHAPTER 1

1 Andreason, N. J. C., Powers, P. S. 'Creativity and psychosis: An examination of conceptual style' *Arch Gen Psychiatry*, 32:70–73, 1973 cited in Goodwin, F. K. & Jamison, K. R. *Manic Depressive Illness* Oxford University Press, New York 1990 p251
2 Barbeau, Clayton C *Dealing with Depression* Franciscan Publications Los Angeles 1987 (video)
3 Stumbles, J. 'Here we go again' in *Voices of the River* Phillip Camela and Fiona Strahan, eds, Disability Employment Action Centre Melbourne 1996
4 Winokur (1969) quoted in F. K. Goodwin, & Jamison, K. R. *Manic Depressive Illness* Oxford University Press New York 1990 p. 48

CHAPTER 2

1 American Psychiatric Association, *Diagnostic and Statistical Manual of Mental Disorders* (4th Edn) American Psychiatric Association Washington DC 1994

2 ibid
3 ibid
4 See Appendix I The Jargon Decoder
5 Goodwin, F. K. and Jamison, K. R. *Manic-Depressive Illness* Oxford University Press New York 1990 p.143
6 ibid
7 ibid
8 Bloch, S. and Singh, B. S. *Understanding Troubled Minds. A guide to mental illness and its treatment* Melbourne University Press Melbourne 1997 p.162
9 Goodwin, F. K. and Jamison, K. R. *Manic-Depressive Illness* Oxford University Press New York 1990 p.449
10 American Psychiatric Association, *Diagnostic and Statistical Manual of Mental Disorders* (3rd Revised Edn) American Psychiatric Association, Washington, DC, cited in Goodwin, F. K. and Jamison, K. R. *Manic-Depressive Illness* Oxford University Press New York 1990 p.109
11 Bloch, S. and Singh, B. S. *Understanding troubled minds. A guide to mental illness and its treatment* Melbourne University Press Melbourne 1997 pp.127–128
12 Goodwin, F. K. and Jamison, K. R. *Manic-Depressive Illness* Oxford University Press New York 1990 p.217
13 ibid
14 In a review of the literature, F. K. Goodwin and K. R. Jamison note the findings of Weissman and colleagues (Weissman M. M., Leaf P. J., Tischler G. L., Blazer D. G., Karno M., Bruce M. L. 'Affective disorders in five US communities' *Psychol Med* 18:141–153 1988a) of a mean cumulative prevalence rate for Bipolar Disorder (defined by a manic episode and thus underestimating by excluding hypomania) as 1.2 per cent. The mean cumulative prevalence of Major Depression was found to be 4.4 per cent in the same study. Source: Goodwin, F. K. and Jamison, K. R. *Manic Depressive Illness* Oxford University Press New York 1990 p.165. By way of comparison, incidence rates for schizophrenia are typically quoted at 1 per cent.
15 Based on ABS estimated resident population of Australia as at September 1996 of 18,348,700.
16 See discussion and review of literature in Goodwin, F. K. and Jamison, K. R. *Manic-Depressive Illness* Oxford University Press New York 1990 pp169–173.
17 Slater, E. and Meyer, A. 'Contributions to a pathography of the musicians: 1. Robert Schumann' *Confin Psychiat* 2:65–94, 1959 quoted in Goodwin, F. K. and Jamison, K. R. *Manic-Depressive Illness* Oxford University Press New York 1990 p.347–349
18 Goodwin, F. K. and Jamison, K. R. *Manic-Depressive Illness* Oxford University Press New York 1990 p.134
19 ibid

20 Angst, J. 'The course of affective disorders: II Typology of bipolar manic-depressive illness.' *Arch Pyschiat Nervenkr* 226:65–73, 1978 cited in Goodwin, F. K. and Jamison, K. R. *Manic-Depressive Illness* Oxford University Press New York 1990 p.139
21 Angst, J. 'Switch from depression to mania, or from mania to depression: Role of psychotropic drugs.' *Psychopharmacol Bull* 23:66–67, 1987 cited in F. K. Goodwin and Jamison K. R. *Manic-Depressive Illness* Oxford University Press New York 1990 p.141
22 ibid
23 American Psychiatric Association, *Diagnostic and Statistical Manual of Mental Disorders* (4th Edn) American Psychiatric Association, Washington DC 1994 p.325
24 Goodwin, F. K. and Jamison, K. R. *Manic-Depressive Illness* Oxford University Press New York 1990 p.534
25 ibid
26 ibid
27 ibid
28 For a more detailed explanation of brain biochemistry and manic depression see Veggeberg, Scott K. *Medication of the Mind* Allen & Unwin Sydney 1996. (First published 1996 Henry Holt & Company, New York.)
29 Parry, B. L. 'Premenstrual and postpartum mood disorders' *Current Opinion in Psychiatry* 9:11–16 1996

CHAPTER 3

1 Goodwin, F. K. and Jamison, K. R. *Manic-Depressive Illness* Oxford University Press New York 1990 pp.46–47
2 'Black mania' coined by Jamison, Kay Redfield in *An Unquiet Mind* Vintage Books New York 1995
3 Moran, Lord Charles *Winston Churchill* Heron Books London 1966 p167
4 Jamison, Kay Redfield *An Unquiet Mind* Vintage Books New York 1995
5 From Kraepelin, 1921 summarised in F. K. Goodwin and K. R. Jamison *Manic-Depressive Illness* Oxford University Press New York 1990 pp.46–47
6 Goodwin, F. K. and Jamison, K. R. *Manic-Depressive Illness* Oxford University Press New York 1990 p.142
7 Leibenluft, E. 'Women with bipolar illness: clinical and research issues' *Am J Psychiatry* 153:2 163–173 1996 Feb
8 Goodwin, F. K. and Jamison, K. R. *Manic-Depressive Illness* Oxford University Press New York 1990 p.143
9 Steiner, Meir 'Premenstrual Dysphoric Disorder—An Update', *General Hospital Psychiatry*, 18:244–250, 1996

10 Roccatagliata G. *A History of Ancient Psychiatry* New York: Greenwood Press, 1986 quoted in Goodwin, F. K. and Jamison, K. R. *Manic-Depressive Illness* Oxford University Press New York 1990 p.562

11 Rosenthal, N.E., Kasper, S., Schulz, P. M. and Wehr, T. A. 'New concepts and developments in seasonal affective disorder' in Thompson, C. and Silverstone, T. (eds) *Seasonal Affective Disorder* London CRC Clinical Neuroscience, in press cited in Goodwin, F. K. and Jamison, K. R. *Manic-Depressive Illness* Oxford University Press New York 1990 p.566

CHAPTER 4

1 Goodwin, F. K. and Jamison, K. R. *Manic-Depressive Illness* Oxford University Press New York 1990

2 Jamison, K. R. *An Unquiet Mind* Vintage Books New York 1995 p.91

3 Millett stated 'Either I was never crazy or I have recovered and can be sane henceforth' in Millett, Kate T*he Loony Bin Trip* Simon & Schuster New York 1990

4 Veggeberg, Scott K. *Medication of the Mind* Allen & Unwin Sydney 1996 (First published Henry Holt and Company, New York 1996) pp.29–30.

5 Goodwin, F. K. and Jamison, K. R. *Manic-Depressive Illness* Oxford University Press New York 1990 p.639

6 ibid

7 ibid

8 Grounds, D. and Holwill, B. for Pharmacotherapy Committee of The Melbourne Clinic *A Guide to Lithium* The Melbourne Clinic, Melbourne July 1994 (brochure)

9 Goodwin, F. K. and Jamison, K. R. *Manic-Depressive Illness* Oxford University Press New York 1990 pp.706–707

10 ibid

11 ibid

12 ibid

13 Grounds, D. and Holwill, B. for Pharmacotherapy Committee of The Melbourne Clinic *A guide to lithium* The Melbourne Clinic, Melbourne July 1994 (brochure)

14 MIMS Australia *MIMS Annual 1996* section 3 p 261

15 This is despite studies that illustrate that newer drugs are less costly when non-drug costs are also taken into account. See for example Davies, A., Langley, P. C., Keks, N. A., Cattas, S. V., Lambert, T. and Schweitzer, I. 'Risperidone versus haloperidol: II. Cost-effectiveness' *Clinical Therapeutics* 20(1): 196–213, 1998 Jan–Feb

16 Personal communications, psychiatrists from Monash University (1997) and the University of Melbourne (1999)

17 MIMS Australia *1999 MIMS Annual* (23rd Edn) MIMS Australia St Leonards NSW 1999
18 Gelenberg A. J. and Hopkins, H. S. 'Antipsychotics in bipolar disorder' *J Clin Pyschiatry* 1996; 57 Suppl 9:49–52
19 Bloch, S. and Singh, B. S. *Understanding Troubled Minds: A Guide to Mental Illness and its treatment*. Melbourne University Press Carlton South 1997 p.270
20 See, for example, Clark, H. M., Berk, M. and Brook, S. 'A randomized controlled single blind study of the efficacy of clonazepam and lithium in the treatment of acute mania.' *Human Psychopharmacology* Vol 12(4) Jul–Aug 1997 325–28
21 MIMS Australia *1999 MIMS Annual* (23rd Edn) MIMS Australia St Leonards NSW 1999
22 Stahl, M. 'How to appease the appetite of psychotropic drugs' *J Clin Psychiatry* 59:10, October 1998
23 Personal communication, Dr David Grounds 2000
24 Human Rights and Equal Opportunity Commission *Human Rights and Mental Illness Report of the National Inquiry into the Human Rights of People with Mental Illness*, Australian Government Publishing Service, Canberra 1993 Vol 1 p.250
25 See Grounds, David and Armstrong, June *Ecstasy & Agony* Lothian Port Melbourne (2nd Edn) 1995 p.75
26 Sidney Bloch and Singh, B. S. *Understanding Troubled Minds: A guide to mental illness and its treatment* Melbourne University Press Carlton South 1997 p.276
27 Cited in James, William *The Varieties of Religious Experience* (first published 1902) Martin E Marty (ed) Penguin Classics 1985 p.137.

CHAPTER 5

1 Ellis A. and Harper, R. *A new guide to rational living* Whilshire Books North Hollywood CA 1975 cited in Bernard, M. E. *Staying Rational in an Irrational World*, McCulloch, Melbourne 1986
2 Bernard, M. E., *Staying Rational in an Irrational World* McCulloch Melbourne 1986 p.24. Used with permission of Dr Albert Ellis
3 Bernard, M. E., *Staying Rational in an Irrational World* McCulloch Melbourne 1986 p.39. Used with permission of Dr Albert Ellis
4 Albert Ellis cited in Bernard, M. E. *Staying Rational in an Irrational World* McCulloch Melbourne 1986 pp.31–32. Used with permission of Dr Albert Ellis
5 Coined by Horney, Karen 1945 cited in Bernard, M. E. *Staying Rational in an Irrational World* McCulloch Melbourne 1986 p.27
6 Bernard, M. E. *Staying Rational in an Irrational World* McCulloch Melbourne 1986 p.29. Used with permission of Dr Albert Ellis
7 ibid
8 ibid

9 See, for example, Burke, J. *Contemporary Approaches to Psychotherapy and Counselling* Brooks/Cole Publishing Co. California 1989
10 From Goodwin, F. K. and Jamison, K. R. *Manic-Depressive Illness* Oxford University Press New York 1990 pp.739–40
11 See, for example Maharishi Mahesh Yogi *The Science of Being and Art of Living* SRM Publications London 1966
12 See, for example, Peter Russell *The TM technique—A skeptic's guide to the TM program* Routledge Keegan Paul Boston 1977 (first published 1976)
13 Geddes and Grosset, *Guide to Natural Healing* David Dale House New Lanark Scotland 1997
14 Mills, S (ed.) *Alternatives in healing* Marshall Editions London 1988 p.24
15 ibid
16 Williams, T. *The Complete Illustrated Guide to Chinese Medicine* Element Books Brisbane 1996

CHAPTER 6

1 Medical Practitioners Board of Victoria *Annual Report 1996* Report to Parliament of Victoria p.17.
2 See, for example, *Mental Health Act (Victoria)* 1986 Section 4(2)(a)
3 The Melbourne Clinic *Your Rights and Responsibilities as a Patient* (brochure) 1996
4 The film *Mr. Jones* (Mike Figgis, director, *Mr. Jones* TriStar Pictures 1993) gives a fairly accurate picture of the use of mechanical restraint.
5 Human Rights and Equal Opportunity Commission *Human Rights and Mental Illness Report of the National Inquiry into the Human Rights of People with Mental Illness* Australian Government Publishing Service Canberra 1993 Vol 1 pp.269–70
6 ibid
7 Personal communications from individuals around Australia including those who use public psychiatric inpatient facilities at The Alfred Hospital and Royal Park Hospital, Melbourne.

CHAPTER 7

1 World Health Organization *Primary Health Care* Report of the International Conference on Primary Health Care Alma-Ata, USSR, 6–12 September 1978 World Health Organization Geneva 1978
2 *Mental Health Act 1990* (New South Wales) S9(1)
3 *Mental Health (Treatment and Care) Act 1994* (Australian Capital Territory) S37
4 *Mental Health Act 1986* (Victoria) S8
5 *Mental Health Act 1996* (Tasmania) S24
6 *Mental Health Act 1993* (South Australia) S12
7 *Mental Health Act 1996* (Western Australia) S26

8 *Mental Health Act* (Northern Territory of Australia) S9(1)
9 *Mental Health Act 1974* (Queensland) S18(2)
10 Department of Human Services circular 'Apprehension of Patients Absent Without Leave' Publication No 97/013 October 1997 states that 'Ambulance transport must be used for all people who have been sedated'.
11 Mental Health Act Victoria 1986 Divisions 1AA and 2; also see Victorian Government Department of Human Services 'Electro-convulsive Therapy—About Your Rights' brochure, 1996
12 Mental Health Legal Centre Inc. (Victoria) Personal communication, 1999

CHAPTER 8

1 It is thought that St Francis, too, may have suffered a form of manic depression. See F. K Goodwin and Jamison, K. R. *Manic-Depressive Illness* Oxford University Press New York 1990 p.362. The prayer often attributed to him is 'Give me the strength to change the things I can change, the serenity to accept the things I can't, and the wisdom to know the difference.'
2 Jamison, Kay Redfield *Touched with Fire: Manic Depressive Illness and the Artistic Temperament* New York Free Press Macmillan 1993
3 Personal communication, Andrew Carter, 1997
4 With thanks to Jon Kroschel, for ideas adapted from his staff training package 'Training for Life' 1999

CHAPTER 9

1 Clarke, Marcus 'Swagmen', *The Peripatetic Philosopher* Melbourne, 1869, quoted in W. Fearn-Wannan *Australian Folklore, a dictionary of Lore, Legends and Popular Allusions* Lansdowne Press Melbourne 1970 p. 440
2 Personal communication, Bernie McCormick 1998
3 Beck, A. T. *Depression—Clinical, Experimental and Theoretical Aspects* Harper & Row (Hoeber Medical Division) 1967 pp.186–207
4 Altman, E. G., Hedeker, D., Peterson, J. L. and Davis, J. M. 'The Altman Self-Rating Mania Scale' *Biol Psychiatry* 1997; 42:948–55
5 Moran, Lord Charles, *Winston Churchill—the struggle for survival 1940–1965* Heron Books London 1966
6 Strahan, S. A. K. *Suicide and Insanity* (2d Edn) London 1894 p.131, cited in William James *Varieties of Religious Experience* (first published Longmans, Green & Co. USA 1902) Penguin Classics USA 1985 p.147
7 Tolstoy, Leo Cited in William James *Varieties of Religious Experience* (first published Longmans, Green & Co. USA 1902) Penguin Classics USA 1985 p.156
8 ibid

CHAPTER 10

1 Stumbles, J. 'And here we go again' in *Voices of the River* Phillip Camela, Fiona Strahan (eds) Disability Employment Action Centre Inc. 1996 pp.57–8
2 Cited by Kroschel, Jon consumer consultant, Melbourne, personal communication 1998
3 Myers-Briggs Type Indicator ©Isabel Briggs Myers 1976.
4 Tait, S. *A user guide to the Disability Discrimination Act* Villamanta Publishing Service Geelong West 1995 p.8
5 Schneider, D. 'When do I disclose? ADA protection and your job' *New Frontiers in Psychosocial Occupational Therapy* The Haworth Press 1998 pp.77–87
6 ibid
7 ibid
8 Tait, S. *A user guide to the Disability Discrimination Act* Villamanta Publishing Service Geelong West 1995 p.21
9 Stumbles, J. 'And here we go again' from *Voices of the River*, Phillip Camela, Fiona Strahan eds. Disability Employment Action Centre Inc. Melbourne 1996 pp.57–8
10 Disability Discrimination Law Advocacy Service Melbourne. Personal communication 1998
11 ibid
12 Personal communication 20 June 1995
13 Personal communication, Dr David Grounds, c1996

CHAPTER 11

1 Richardson, Henry Handel *Maurice Guest* (first published William Heinemann 1908) Virago London 1981 p.293
2 *The Age* Melbourne 27 September 1997 p.A31
3 Fitzroy Legal Service *The Law Handbook 1996* Melbourne 1996 p.179
4 Fitzroy Legal Service *The Law Handbook 1996* Melbourne 1996 pp.179–180
5 ibid
6 Hartley, Anne *Debt free* Doubleday Sydney 1992
7 According to *Human Rights and Mental Illness* (the 'Burdekin report'), many life insurance policies represent areas in which people with mental illness encounter 'unjustified discrimination'. The Inquiry was told that insurance companies frequently impose loadings, or even exclusions, on people who have (or have had) a mental illness. 'Witnesses considered these ... out of keeping with the true risk ... the type of illness, its severity, its prognosis or its consequences for longevity or for income-earning capacity'. Human Rights and Equal Opportunity Commission *Human Rights and Mental Illness. Report of the National Inquiry into the Human Rights of People with Mental Illness*, Canberra, Australian Government Publishing Service 1993 p.449

8 See for example 'Will Kit', Australian Will Company PO Box 202 East Bentleigh Victoria 3165

CHAPTER 12

1 Pomeroy, E. and Trainor, J. *Families of people with mental illness: Current dilemmas and strategies for change* Canadian Mental Health Association 1991 p.31

CHAPTER 13

1 Sayce, Liz 'Parenting as a civil right: supporting service users who choose to have children' in A. Weir and A. Douglas *Child Protection and Adult Mental Health* Butterworth-Heinemann Oxford 1999
2 See for example S. Lancaster 'Being there: How parental mental illness can affect children' in *Children of parents with mental illness* V. Cowling (ed.) ACER Press Melbourne 1999.
3 See, for example:
Cowling, V. 1996a 'Meeting the support needs of families with dependent children where the parent has a mental illness' *Family Matters* No 45 Spring/Summer 1996 pp.22–5;
Cowling, V. 1996b *Children of parents experiencing major mental illness* Stage II(b) Report on interviews with thirteen parents, 11 July 1996 University of Melbourne;
Wang A. and Goldschmidt, V. V. 'Interviews with psychiatric inpatients about professional intervention with regard to their children' *Acta Psychiatr Scand* 1996; 93: 57–61;
Cowling, V. (ed.) *Children of parents with mental illness* ACER Press Melbourne 1999;
Weir A. and Douglas, A. *Child Protection and Adult Mental Health* Butterworth-Heinemann Oxford 1999
4 See, for example, The Melbourne Consumer Consultants' Group Inc. *Do you mind? The ultimate exit survey: Survivors of psychiatric services speak out* Melbourne Consumer Consultants' Group Inc Melbourne 1997 p.45
5 Human Rights and Equal Opportunity Commission *Human Rights and Mental Illness. Report of the National Inquiry into the Human Rights of People with Mental Illness* Canberra Australian Government Publishing Service 1993 p.499
6 See, for example, Cowling, V. (ed.) *Children of parents with mental illness* ACER Press Melbourne 1999
7 Kelly, Madeleine 'Approaching the last resort: a parent's view' in V. Cowling (ed.) *Children of parents with mental illness* ACER Press Melbourne 1999. See also Liz Sayce, 'Parenting as a civil right: supporting service users who choose to have children' in A. Weir and A. Douglas *Child Protection and Adult Mental Health—conflict of interest?* Butterworth-Heinemann Oxford 1999.

8 Jamison, K. R. *An Unquiet Mind* Vintage Books New York 1996, p.193. See also Goodwin, F. K. and Jamison, K. R. *Manic-Depressive Illness* Oxford, New York 1990 p.366
9 Grounds, D. and Armstrong, J. *Ecstasy and Agony* Lothian Melbourne (first published 1992, 2nd Edn 1995) p.140
10 Goodwin, F. K. and Jamison, K. R. *Manic-Depressive Illness* Oxford University Press New York 1990 p.397

CHAPTER 14

1 Backhouse, Halcyon (ed.) St. John of the Cross *The Dark Night of the Soul* Hodder & Stoughton Christian Classics London 1988 p.14
2 James, William *The Varieties of Religious Experience* First pub 1902 Martin E Marty (ed) Penguin Classics 1985
3 ibid p.83
4 ibid p.91
5 ibid p.128
6 Griffin, Graeme *Death and the church: problems and possibilities* Dove Communications Melbourne 1978 p.54
7 James, William *The Varieties of Religious Experience* First pub 1902 Martin E Marty (ed) Penguin Classics 1985 p.136
8 ibid p.167
9 Backhouse, Halcyon (ed.) St. John of the Cross, *The Dark Night of the Soul*, Hodder & Stoughton Christian Classics London 1988 p.14
10 American Psychiatric Association, *Diagnostic and Statistical Manual of Mental Disorders* Fourth Edition, American Psychiatric Association Washington DC 1994
11 Freud, Sigmund 'Obsessive actions and religious practices' in J. Strachey (ed. and trans.) *The standard edition of the complete psychological works of Sigmund Freud* (Vol 1) Hogarth Press London 1966 cited in Lukoff, D., Turner, R. and Lu, F. 'Transpersonal Psychology Research Review: Psychoreligious Dimensions of Healing' *Journal of Transpersonal Psychology* 1992 Vol 24 No 1 p.41
12 Bernard, M *Staying Rational in an Irrational World* McCullough Publishing Melbourne 1986 pp.260–261
13 Jung, C *Memories, Dreams, Reflections* Fount Glasgow 1977 (first published 1961) pp.160–162
14 Lukoff D. and Everest, H. Everest 'Myths in mental illness' *Journal of Transpersonal Psychology* 1985 17(2), 123–53 cited in D. Lukoff, R. Turner and F. Lu, 'Transpersonal Psychology Research Review: Psychoreligious Dimensions of Healing' *Journal of Transpersonal Psychology* 1992 Vol 24, No 1
15 Lukoff, D., Turner, R. and Lu, F. 'Transpersonal Psychology Research Review: Psychoreligious Dimensions of Healing' in *Journal of Transpersonal Psychology* 1992 Vol 24, No 1 pp.45–46

16 Taylor, M. and Abrams, R. 'Acute mania: clinical and genetic study of responders and nonresponders to treatments' *Archives of General Psychiatry* 1975 Vol 32 cited in Watkins, J. *Hearing Voices* Hill of Content Melbourne 1998 p.67
17 Winokur, G., Clayton, P. J. and Reich, T. *Manic Depressive Illness* St Louis: CV Mosby 1967 cited in Goodwin, F. K. and Jamison, K. R. *Manic-Depressive Illness* Oxford New York 1990 p.361
18 Lukoff, D. 'The Diagnosis of mystical experiences with psychotic features' *Journal of Transpersonal Psychology* 1985 Vol 17 No 2 p.156.
19 Laing, R. D. *The Politics of Experience* New York 1967 Ballantyne cited in Lukoff (1985), op. cit.
20 Lukoff, D 'The Diagnosis of Mystical Experiences with Psychotic Features' *Journal of Transpersonal Psychology* 1985, Vol 17, No 2, p.156.
21 Ibid., p.168.
22 Ibid., p.170.
23 Lukoff, D., Lu, F. and Turner, R. 'Toward a more culturally sensitive DSM-IV. Psychoreligious and psychospiritual problems' *Journal of Nervous and Mental Disease* Vol 180 No1 Sept. 1992
24 American Psychiatric Association, *Diagnostic and Statistical Manual of Mental Disorders* Fourth edition, American Psychiatric Association Washington DC 1994
25 Lukoff, D., Turner, R. and Lu, F. 'Transpersonal Psychology Research Review: Psychoreligious Dimensions of Healing.' *Journal of Transpersonal Psychology* 1992 Vol 24 No 1
26 Fox, Matthew *The Coming of the Cosmic Christ* HarperCollins New York 1988 p.41
27 Griffin, Graeme *Death and the church: problems and possibilities* Dove Communications Melbourne 1978 p.55
28 Jones, Alexander (ed.) *The Jerusalem Bible* Darton, Longman & Todd, London 1968
29 St. John of the Cross, *Ascent of Mount Carmel*, cited in Watkins, J. *Hearing Voices* Hill of Content Melbourne 1998 p.188
30 ibid p.189
31 See Watkins, J. *Hearing Voices* Hill of Content Melbourne 1998 pp.189–191

CONCLUSION

1 With apologies to Robert Lowell (1917–1977), whose poem 'Since 1939' from *Day by Day* (Farrar, Straus and Giraux New York 1977) gave us the vernacular: 'if we see a light at the end of the tunnel,/it's the light of an oncoming train' source F. K. Goodwin, and K. R. Jamison, *Manic-Depressive Illness* Oxford New York 1990 p.19

APPENDIX I

1 I have attempted to give readers the most useful colloquial meanings and have also referred to the *New Shorter Oxford Dictionary* 1993.

2 Bloch, S & Singh, B.S. *Understanding troubled minds* Melbourne University Press Carlton South 1997 p54

INDEX